Gut Feelings

Gut Feelings

Healing the Shame-Fuelled Relationship Between What You Eat and How You Feel

DR WILL COLE
with Gretchen Lidicker

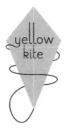

First published in the United States in 2023 by Rodale Books,
An imprint of Random House,
A division of Penguin Random House LLC, New York
First published in Great Britain in 2023 by Yellow Kite
An imprint of Hodder & Stoughton
An Hachette UK company

1

A CIP catalogue record for this title is available from the British Library

Hardback ISBN 9781399724173
eBook ISBN 9781399724111

Typeset in Minion Pro by Andrea Lau

Printed and bound in Great Britain by Clays Ltd, Elcograf S.p.A.

Hodder & Stoughton policy is to use papers that are natural, renewable and recyclable
products and made from wood grown in sustainable forests. The logging and
manufacturing processes are expected to conform to the environmental regulations of the
country of origin.

Hodder & Stoughton Ltd
Carmelite House
50 Victoria Embankment
London EC4Y 0DZ

www.yellowkitebooks.co.uk

Amber, Solomon, and Shiloh:
"When my body dies, my soul will still be yours.
Nothing is lost. Only changed."

CONTENTS

FOREWORD

Gut feelings. Is there anything else more important than these guiding pings from our deepest intuition? Dr. Will Cole, a colleague and friend of mine, has written a paradigm-shifting way to truly understand the inherent and foundational connection between our body and mind. The pages of this book offer a new way of thinking about your gut as a second brain and will open you up to an entirely new way of taking control of your health. By the end of this book, you'll feel fully empowered to create true and lasting wellness for both your body and mind.

Today so many of us feel depressed, anxious, and completely apathetic toward life. With more and more access to mental healthcare, the question becomes: *Is there something deeper going on here?* In *Gut Feelings,* Dr. Cole drops mind-blowing education on just how deep it goes. He takes you on a journey to the root cause of many common symptoms and chronic health issues in a scientific yet incredibly accessible way.

Dr. Cole shares the science of inflammation and gut issues, like bacterial overgrowth and leaky gut, that can lead to depression, mood swings, and other mental health symptoms. His explanation of the underlying source of many common symptoms offers the missing piece from traditional medical practitioners, who focus primarily on symptom management. Understanding the factors that contribute to your daily health struggles will offer many of you relief from a lifetime of unanswered questions and may even bring up deeper emotions from those of us who may feel that, for the first time, *a doctor finally gets me.*

Most notably, Dr. Cole makes the connection between emotions and health problems that stem from what he calls *Shameflammation*. As a holistic psychologist who now runs a global membership community, I have witnessed the role emotions, especially stress, play in the physical wellness (or illness) of individuals everywhere. I have also seen innumerable instances of different emotional struggles stemming from physical imbalances caused by nutritional and lifestyle choices. I can only hope that this book gets in the hands of every mental health professional to better equip them with more information about the mind-body relationship.

I believe that the best healers are practitioners of their craft, and Dr. Will Cole is a true practitioner. His experience working with thousands of people around the world translates into a depth of wisdom that is unparalleled. He works daily to embody his own mind-body wellness and graciously shares this information and these transformational tools with innumerable others across his social media platforms. He is truly an inspirational guide pointing us all to a path toward a healthier and happier life.

I am so grateful this life-changing book landed in your hands. The information presented will shift how you think, how you eat, and, ultimately, how you exist in the world. The practical tools—especially the 21-Day Gut-Feeling Plan—will show you just how much the food you eat daily truly does impact your mood and health. By the end of this book, you will have the information you need and a road map to change who you are at your core (*literally!*).

Spend time with this book. Take notes if you want to. Then, most important, begin to put these things into practice. Your body and mind will thank you.

—Nicole LePera, PhD

Thought for Food:
The Gut-Feeling Connection

It's been said that gut feelings are guardian angels. They provide that deep-knowing, discerning intuition that has guided and protected you throughout your life. They are the ineffable inner sixth sense with its still-small voice, giving you the visceral understanding that it has your back. "Gut feelings," "trust your gut," and "gut instinct" are all sentiments with ancient origins. Somehow humanity has always known that the gut is the seat of the soul; and today, in our modern world, we know that at our very creation, when we were in our mother's womb, our gut and brain were formed from the same tissue, inextricably woven together for the rest of our life in sacred union.

Your brain-gut connection is a galaxy of brilliance, a cerebral garden of wonderment and dreams. The vast confluence of synapses and neurons contained within your mental masterpiece could stretch farther than the moon. Your gut is equally vast, with more bacteria than you have human cells, more in number than the stars in the sky. In fact, the trillions of cells that make up your brain and body were formed from the same carbon, oxygen, and nitrogen as the stars that shone brightly billions of years ago. You are literally stardust personified—the cosmos incarnate.

If you've ever gotten that quick thrill of butterflies on a first date or felt the ache of your stomach dropping when you received bad news, you've already experienced the gut-feeling connection in real life. There's no way around it: The bidirectional relationship between your gut and feelings is intimately at play every single day of your life. These gut feelings can contain innumerable inspirations for hope, healing, and self-protection, but they can also be tainted with shame, anger, and fear, becoming the single biggest saboteur of your health. When these gut feelings work against us, they can end up sabotaging our health and creating very real physical health imbalances. From autoimmune conditions to anxiety, blood sugar issues to brain fog, and hormone imbalances to heart problems—whatever it is that ails you, your gut-feeling connection is playing a role.

In the Western world, we like to separate mental health from physical health, but the truth is that mental health *is* physical health. Our brain is part of our body—and there isn't a single health condition out there that doesn't require us to heal both. As a functional medicine doctor, I talk a lot about how the gut is the center of human health. It controls not just our digestion but also our immune system, metabolism, and mood. It's not only that physical health imbalances will impact you mentally and emotionally—what's going on in your inner psychological world will impact every physiological system and cell of your body, and it does all this through your gut-feeling connection.

When I bring this connection up to my patients, some of them are totally open to addressing it and are willing to rethink the way they approach physical health. Other times, I'm met with some resistance. If this is you, I get it. Addressing the effect of our emotional world on our body can make us feel out of control. Why? Because to do it, we must admit that achieving optimal health isn't necessarily a straight path, a cut-and-dried mission, or a quantitative equation of X hours of sleep + Y ounces of leafy greens + Z workouts a week.

I think we can all admit that there's a part of us that would like health to be this way: *Tell us the rules and we'll follow them! Give us a checklist of habits for good health, and we'll tick them off one by one!* Many of us would love nothing more than a clear bulleted list of the things we need to do to stay healthy and happy. Checking in on our "inner world" and cultivating a deeper relationship with ourselves and our bodies was not exactly what we had in mind.

Not to mention, in a world where our to-do lists are long, distractions are endless, juice bars and fitness studios are on every block, and supplement cabinets are overflowing (who else has a supplement graveyard somewhere in their house?), addressing our whole-body health is even more critical. Why? Because many of us can go from one wellness practice and modality to the next without acknowledging the effect of our mental and emotional world and our health. This can leave us in a cycle of suffering, spending, and wondering what the heck we're doing wrong. Even worse, most health experts, nutrition books, and diet plans focus just on physical health. While the world we live in today may be overflowing with health and wellness advice, very little of it truly addresses both the body and the mind.

That's where this book comes in. In the following pages, I'll provide a framework for you to better understand the effect of your emotional world on your physical world and vice versa. As you turn the following pages, you'll learn how to nourish not only your physical health, but also your mental health. There is both a science and an art to healing your gut-feeling connection. This book is holding both in harmony so that you can reclaim your wellness.

This book is different from anything I've ever written. As you make your way through the pages ahead, you won't find strict recommendations for what to do and when or a list of foods to eliminate and a list of foods to eat for the 21 days. Instead, you'll find something unexpected. Together, we'll set off on a journey of grace and lightness, with many twists and turns, that will help us discover how to live our healthiest and happiest life. Think of this book as a call to action to slow down, breathe, and allow your body to do what it does best—heal.

Are you ready to step into the unknown?

CHAPTER 1

As Above, So Below

The Bidirectional Relationship Between Your Physical and Emotional World

If you raised an eyebrow (or two) when you read the introduction to this book, I'm not surprised. You might even doubt that there *is* an emotional side to health. To that I would say: One, keep reading, and two, keep an open mind. After years of working with people all around the world in my functional medicine telehealth clinic, I've seen the emotional side of health affect so many people. As a functional medicine doctor, I'm trained to look at the person as a whole instead of seeing the body as separate unrelated parts like in the conventional medicine world. I often collaborate with conventional physicians, therapists, and holistic practitioners to organize the best protocols healthcare has to offer for my patients (there's a reason why functional medicine is also known as *integrative medicine*), serving as a prover-bial "wellness quarterback" for my patients. A person's mental, emotional, and spiritual world is not just part of that overall holistic picture, it's the critical piece.

Later on, we'll dive into the nitty-gritty, granular reasons why our physical and emotional lives are intertwined. For example, we'll talk about how gut bacteria can influence our mood and how stress can cause physiological changes that sabotage our health. But we're not there just yet! Right now, I want to zoom out and talk about the practical everyday ways this gut-feeling connection reveals itself in our lives.

How the Physical Impacts the Emotional

From years of clinical experience in nutrition and lifestyle medicine, I know that physical health factors are more than capable of impacting your emotional world. You might be shaking your head, thinking, *Well, of course, Dr. Cole—nobody likes to be sick, in pain, or have a disease!* While it's true that having a chronic health condition or being sick can be a difficult emotional experience, I'm not necessarily talking about the emotional hardship of a diagnosed disease or the trauma of an acute illness, even though this certainly adds to the cycle of stress and health problems. Instead, I'm talking about the less obvious physical health imbalances—like chronic inflammation or gut-health microbiome imbalances—that can more subtly sabotage our emotional health day after day, year after year. This physical-emotional connection is insidious because it's often ignored by the conventional healthcare world, which treats mental health and emotional health as if the brain exists completely unconnected to the rest of the body. And yet it seems like every single day, mental health issues like anxiety, depression, or PTSD are connected to physical health factors, like diet, inflammation levels, or the status of the gut microbiome, further proving that the physical and emotional world has always been and always will be intertwined.

Just to give you a few examples:

- More and more studies are asserting that depression may be caused by chronic systemic inflammation in the body and showing that anti-inflammatory foods reduce symptoms of depression.
- Problems with the gut, such as yeast or bacterial overgrowth, often present themselves in the form of mood swings, anxiety, and persistent food cravings. When a patient comes in with any of these brain issues, the gut is the first thing I look at.
- Studies have suggested that inadequate immune system control and inflammation may raise the risk of developing PTSD after a trauma.[1]
- Studies show that even mild dehydration can be linked to anxiety, tension, and

mood disturbance, demonstrating that something as simple as drinking more water and supporting electrolyte balance could improve mental health.[2]

- Here's one you probably already know: A more sedentary lifestyle has been linked to an increased risk of anxiety and depression. But did you also know that exercise has been shown to be as effective if not more effective at reducing depression than prescription antidepressants? It's true.[3]

If you've ever been told that mental health issues have nothing to do with your physical health, you're not alone. But I'm here to tell you that the connection between the two is all too real and couldn't be more relevant to your health and healing.

How the Emotional Influences the Physical

Now that we've established how physical health influences emotional health, let me ask you a question: Have you ever eaten a perfectly "healthy" meal and ended up bloated and with stomach pains? Often that's because you sat down stressed and anxious, ate while you were distracted or still in fight-or-flight mode, and then went back to your hectic day without a moment of peace or stillness. Just like food, our thoughts and emotions have the power to make us feel terrible or fuel our bodies with vibrant health. In my years practicing functional medicine, I've seen any number of the following:

- I've seen patients with chronic digestive issues cut virtually every "trigger" food out of their diet but see their digestive health continue to decline because of chronic stress.
- I've seen patients try every exercise and diet that exists but continue to hold on to weight because their body is in fight or flight from an abusive relationship or past trauma.
- I've seen patients try every conventional and natural treatment to quell their

autoimmune condition, trying to force it into submission instead of taking a break from their hyperintense job or exercise routine.

- I have many patients who don't know which came first—the digestive problem or the depression, the autoimmunity or the anxiety, the migraines or the mood disorder.

On the other end . . .

- I've seen patients quit a toxic job and completely reverse health conditions that had been getting worse for years.
- I've seen patients start meditating and investing in stress reduction and end up healing from chronic fatigue, hormone imbalances, inflammatory disorders, and so much more.
- I've seen patients start therapy and end up healing not just from anxiety and depression but also from migraines, allergies, IBS, psoriasis, acne—the list goes on ad infinitum.
- I've seen patient after patient break down in our consultations online, admitting that they feel sad, desperate, ignored, neglected, angry, or frustrated, and then report that they feel physical relief almost immediately just from being heard and letting their pent-up, suppressed emotions out.

When I see any of these patients going through experiences like the ones I mentioned above, the deeply mysterious, emotional nature of these situations always strikes me. Despite our best efforts to control certain aspects of our health by taking our supplements and medications and eating all the "right" things, if we don't address the emotional component of our health, we can never truly heal. These are just a few of the many, many moments over the years that have made me a true believer in the bidirectional relationship between physical and emotional health.

Shameflammation

In my book *The Inflammation Spectrum*, I describe chronic inflammation as a smol-dering fire within, a fire that goes largely unnoticed until it turns into any number of health problems. Well, throughout my years of treating patients and helping them get their bodies and minds back to vibrant health, I've seen the way that neg-ative thoughts and emotions can subtly and systematically sabotage health, in much the same way as inflammation can. In fact, I see this phenomenon of emotional suffering causing physical suffering so often that I decided to give it its own name: *Shameflammation*.

Shameflammation is present in every single one of us to some degree, and it can make us feel overwhelmed, anxious, hopeless, aimless, and totally disconnected from our intuition. It can be both the underlying cause and result of chronic health conditions—it's often the one thing standing between us and optimal health. Shameflammation can make us feel like we're constantly swimming upstream and at war with our bodies. Thoughts and emotions are like nutrients for your head, heart, and soul; and unfortunately, many of us have been feeding ourselves junk food for a long, long time.

So, now let's answer the question I know a lot of you are asking yourselves: *Why shame? Out of all the negative emotions in this world, why do we use shame for the term that represents the negative impact of our emotional world on the physical?* Over the years, I've learned that shame is perhaps the strongest, most damaging negative emotion of all. Brené Brown, a renowned shame and vulnerability researcher, says that "shame is lethal" and explains that shame affects all of us and profoundly shapes the way we interact in the world.[4]

After years of consulting patients with all types of health struggles, I can say that nowhere is shame more at play than when it comes to our bodies and our health. It's often a huge barrier to healing. Let me ask you this: When something goes awry with your body or health, big or small, how do you feel? The answer is probably a mixture of anger, fear, and maybe even some embarrassment, right? That sounds a whole lot like shame to me. The common thread between many emotions, especially those surrounding our body and our health, is often shame. Research shows that, as humans, we feel a lot of health-related shame and that shame can have a significant impact on our ability to stay healthy, heal from illness, and make healthy choices. Why? Because any type of shame—whether it's related to food, our body, or a health condition—makes us feel unworthy of the vibrant health we crave, cutting us off at our knees as we try to get there. According to shame experts, shame exists on a spectrum, ranging from self-consciousness or embarrassment to a deep sense of inadequacy and fear, but these feelings all tell us one thing at the end of the day—that we don't deserve that healthy and happy life.

Unfortunately, despite knowing that shame affects our health in big and small ways, we don't know all that much else due to a lack of research in this area. In one fascinating study, researchers posited that the impact of shame on our health "is unacknowledged, under-researched, and undertheorised in the context of health and medicine." They go on to say that shame can have a significant impact on health, illness, and health-related behaviors and that shame's influence can be described only as "insidious, pervasive, and pernicious."[5] Pretty strong language, isn't it? It is, but it's also true. Your healing can't shine when it's soaked in shame.

And then, there's the other half of the word *Shameflammation*, the part that includes *inflammation*. Inflammation is a topic I speak about a lot as a functional medicine practitioner. Inflammation is actually a lifesaving biological process that was expertly created to help protect you from harm. When your inflammatory response is working the way it was designed, your body will launch a protective inflammatory response when you encounter a pathogen, such as the flu virus or a harmful bacteria like *Staphylococcus* or *Streptococcus*—and it will send inflammatory immune cells to the area to take down the threat, kill it, and then return your body to a state of calm. Inflammation also responds to injury. Have you ever broken a bone or sprained an ankle and noticed that it gets red, inflamed, and painful? That's your inflammatory response rushing to the area to keep the hurt from spreading and to encourage you to rest so the area has time to heal.

But this is true only when inflammation is acting the way it was designed to work. And for many of us, this is unfortunately not the case. Instead, many of us deal with chronic inflammation. This chronic inflammation is caused by a whole list of factors such as toxins in our environment, too much sugar in our diet, and a sedentary lifestyle. Chronic inflammation can also be triggered by stress, shame, and difficult emotional experiences. And when shame-triggered inflammation is high over a long period of time, it can contribute to disease. One particularly damaging pro-inflammatory protein that spikes during times of mental-emotional stress is something called *interleukin-6* (*IL-6* for short). An interesting study published in the journal *Brain, Behavior, and Immunity* looked at the relationship between mental stress, our brains, and inflammation. The researchers had forty-one healthy adult participants do something that most of us sweat at just the thought of: math. As if that wasn't scary enough, they had the test subjects do it in front of a group of judges plus deliver a five-minute public speech. Afterward, the researchers took blood samples from the participants. They found that the longer they did math or spoke in public, the higher their IL-6 (inflammation) levels were. In fact, while you might think that the levels of inflammation would go down after the participants had been doing it for a while, that wasn't the case. On the second day of public speaking and problem-solving, stress and IL-6 levels spiked even higher than on the first.[6]

But what the researchers discovered next was also astounding. It turned out that the group with the highest measured levels of self-compassion before the study— the ones who had the highest levels of acceptance of themselves—had the lowest IL-6 (inflammation) response to the stress.

This is a powerful message. Stress, shame, inflammation, Shameflammation— it's all inevitable to some degree. But our relationship with ourselves in the present moment contributes to whether the challenges we face flood our body with inflammation or are met with calming balance, allowing our body to thrive. This is why so much of taming Shameflammation, which we'll learn about in future chapters, has to do with self-compassion. Self-compassion and a sense of being your biggest cheerleader should always be the underlying cause of anything you do for your health and wellness. Why? You can't heal a body you hate.

Now, I know that there's no such thing as a life without stress. We will all face stressors of one type or another, whether they involve our finances, our health, our education, our relationships, or our family. But that's not where our negative emotional experiences begin and end. As humans, we also experience deeper, more complex, and more intense feelings that can also affect our health.

The bottom line is that shame is ever-present in our lives and ever-relevant when it comes to our relationship with ourselves and our health. When I'm consulting with my patients from my functional medicine telehealth clinic, often the intersection between shame and inflammation—Shameflammation—is what stands between them and their healing.

Is Shameflammation Sabotaging Your Health?

So, I know you are all wondering what signs indicate that your emotional world is affecting your physical health. The first sign is that you're struggling with conditions like anxiety, depression, PTSD, or another trauma disorder. That said, the effects of shame can go far beyond mental health. When I'm consulting with patients online, I look for the following signs and symptoms and always flag them as a reason to dig deeper into their inner world:

- Physical pain that can't be explained or treated
- A hormone imbalance
- A disconnection from your intuition, especially when it comes to food and wellness
- Brain fog and light-headedness
- Autoimmune conditions
- Heart palpitations (the feeling that your heart is racing)
- A chronic health issue that is exacerbated or triggered by stress
- Chronic fatigue that can't be explained
- A chronically stiff neck or back
- Constipation or diarrhea even after making dietary changes
- Extreme tiredness or fatigue, with normal lab results and no clear explanation

- Insomnia
- Low libido or problems with sexual performance
- Mood changes that seem unrelated to what's going on in your life
- Chronic bloating or gas despite making dietary changes
- A chronic health condition that developed after a traumatic experience
- Weight gain or loss without a clear explanation
- Change in appetite and nausea
- A lack of motivation to make lifestyle changes
- Feeling like you're constantly swimming upstream
- Being overwhelmed by all the nutrition and health advice in the world
- Constantly comparing your diet and lifestyle, your health and body, to what you see around you
- A feeling of aimlessness or hopelessness when it comes to health and nutrition

Taming Shameflammation with the Gut-Feeling Lifestyle Plan

So, how do you tame Shameflammation? Regardless of how big a role it's playing in our lives, getting Shameflammation under control requires us to get our gut-feeling connection back in sync—and we can do this by focusing not only on the foods that are kind to our gut but also on the practices that are friendly to our mind. When we tackle Shameflammation from both the gut side and the feeling side, we can restore that gut-brain connection and stop swimming upstream.

In many instances, the antidote to this Shameflammation is a process of slowing down, getting still, and reconnecting with yourself. When you do this, it begins a beautiful process of shifting and realigning the paradigm: You begin to view health and healing as an investment in the body and the mind and understand the connection between them. That journey to sustainable wellness doesn't happen overnight, but it's so worth it. I've always aimed to imbue my nutrition and lifestyle plans with grace, ease, and self-love. And in this book, I'm taking it a step further with the 21-Day Gut-Feeling Plan, which is infused with flexibility and simplicity to quiet the noise and get you back in touch with those invaluable gut feelings.

At the core of the Gut-Feeling Plan is addressing your gut-feeling connection from a holistic point of view. The goal of this book is to learn that wellness is a sacred art, and you are the masterpiece. Everything I'll teach you throughout the course of this book about the body and mind comes together in the lifestyle plan, which takes you on a 21-day journey to reset your gut health, restore your energy, and reboot the connection between physical and emotional health. So what does that look like in practice?

The Gut-Feeling Plan is not a detox, cleanse, or elimination diet. It's something that can be completed anytime, anywhere, and maintained for your entire life. It's designed to be flexible and fun. The Gut-Feeling Plan is a new way of thinking about wellness—one that focuses on what's going on in your head and heart as much as on what's filling your plate. For 21 days, I'll take you through a series of practices and lessons I've collected over the years that have had a huge impact on my patients and my own health, too.

Each day will be divided into two parts: gut and feelings. Every day, there will be one tip or action item for each equally important facet of health. Some of the tips or action items involve reflecting on your diet, cravings, or habits around food—and I will suggest changes you can make that will help you optimize health and happiness—and others are practices that I've seen help my patients and followers optimize the gut-feeling connection. For the gut, this could be anything from trying out a gut-healing food to tracking your water or sugar intake to experimenting with leaving a fourteen-hour gap between dinner and breakfast the next day. The feeling items will be anything from gratitude practices to a breathing exercise to a bath.

The Gut-Feeling Plan is all about reflection and experimentation. As you move through it, I offer you the opportunity to make changes to your diet and lifestyle, but what those changes look like, how drastic they are, and whether you do them for that single day or continue with that practice for the rest of the 21 days (or even beyond!) is up to you. The exercises in the 21-Day Gut-Feeling Plan are meant to inspire playful experimentation and celebration of your body and mind.

Proverbial Food Fights: Letting Your Food Peace FLAG Fly

It's no surprise that I'm an advocate for many diverse wellness practices, especially those that are founded on the idea of food as medicine. That said, a big part of writing this book for me was reflecting on the ways that wellness culture has inadvertently contributed to a distorted gut-feeling connection and Shameflammation. One big factor that I know plays a role is the sheer number of mixed messages about healthy living coming from all directions. Too much advice draws hard-and-fast rules about what's healthy and what's not, leaving us feeling like failures if we don't follow it word for word. This inevitably leads to frustration, stress, and dread—and you know what that means: Shameflammation. We've given ourselves labels such as paleo, keto, vegan, low carb, vegetarian or carnivore, trapping ourselves in boxes and leaving ourselves little room to listen to our own intuition or gut feelings about what our bodies and minds really need to heal. But here's the truth: There is no best method that holds the secret to perfect health for all humans, and anyone telling you different is perpetuating ideas from a toxic diet culture that we should all look the same and eat the same to be healthy and happy—as if humans are anything but wonderfully unique. If we all ate and exercised exactly the same way, we would still all look, weigh, and feel very differently. We are all individuals, and even the "healthiest" food for one person may not be the best for you. Conversely, food, exercise, or wellness practices that don't make you feel great may work just fine for someone else. As we move through this book, I'll be pointing out other ways to free yourself from this linear thinking and to tackle this often-ignored cause of Shameflammation. Bio-individuality is the heart of functional medicine and human health.

As you'll experience when you get to the plan, I designed the 21-Day Gut-Feeling Lifestyle Plan to help you explore a balanced approach to food and eating. This plan teaches us that we can hold two competing thoughts in our brain at the same time—that eating healthy can improve our health but also that stressing about food can sabotage our health just the same—and find a food solution that still makes sense for us. If you want to feel your best, you must find a way to strike a balance between honoring the physical without sabotaging the emotional and honoring the emotional without sabotaging the physical. Looking after both sides is the foundation of the Gut-Feeling Plan—it aims to create a solid foundation of nutrition that gives your body the tools it needs to function at its very best. It does this by promoting the consumption of nutrient-dense foods healthy for your gut and your brain while helping you identify and reflect on the foods and practices that might be causing problems.

The nutrition part of the Gut-Feeling Plan is founded upon four key principles:

- Flexibility: This means being open-minded about learning which foods your body loves and make you feel great. It means not being rigid but embracing and evolving with curiosity.
- Lightness: You can allow your thoughts and emotions around food and wellness to pass through you instead of holding on to them and identifying with them. If something didn't work for you, let it go.
- Awareness: By using food as a meditation and eating more mindfully, you will learn which foods make you feel great and which ones don't. Avoiding foods that make you feel physically inflamed, bloated, fatigued, or any form of yucky isn't restrictive. It's self-respect. Ask yourself, "Does this food make me feel great or not?" Focus on foods that make you feel great.
- Grace: If eating the food—even the food that didn't make you feel great afterward—was worth it, quit shaming yourself and give yourself and this process some grace and move on. Shame is worse than any junk food. If it wasn't worth it, then you'll grow in awareness for the next time. You are learning to love feeling great more than you thought you wanted that food that made you feel bad.

In other words, let your Food Peace **FLAG** fly!

Beyond that, the plan is about approaching nutrition and wellness from a place of self-love and celebration, not from a need to maintain a "perfect" diet or lifestyle, which will end up sabotaging your gut-feeling connection more than helping it. In other words, you build that solid foundation, and then the rest of your focus is on being satisfied and happy with the choices you've made.

Before we dive into the plan itself and get to addressing the gut-feeling connection, let's dive into the gut and our feelings individually so we can understand how they are connected and play a role in our health.

CHAPTER 2

Gut

The Physiology of the Second Brain

Have you ever heard the saying, "The gut is the second brain"? Whether this is the first time you're reading those words or the thousandth, they seem to become truer every day. When you feel the sting of rejection, a pang of loneliness, or that little "nudge-nudge" of intuition about something or someone, it's not just your imagination that you feel it in the gut. All emotions—anything from sadness to excitement to fear—can lead to changes in the functioning of the gut. The gut and the brain communicate directly back and forth in a very real way. Have you ever looked at a delicious plate of food and immediately found your stomach growling? Have you ever felt nervous and lost your appetite? Have you ever pulled an all-nighter and craved sugar the whole next day? That's just your gut being your good ol' second brain.

For the past several years, scientists have been able to deepen our understanding of this link, drawing connections between mental health conditions, like anxiety and depression, and the gut. In this chapter, we'll be diving into the magnificent and mysterious world of the gut, including what's new in research on the gut-brain connection and how the ins and outs of the gut affect our health every single day. And we'll be starting at the very center of it all—the gut microbiome.

The Microbiome and Your Mood

<>><><><><><><><><><><><><><><><><><><><><><><><><><><><><><><><><><><><><><><><><><><>

I'd be surprised if you didn't know a thing or two about the gut microbiome already. You may have heard something from a friend or family member or read something on the news about the benefits of probiotic supplements for gut health, weight loss, or bloating. There's a good chance you're well acquainted with the idea that the gut microbiome plays a role in your health.

If you're new to the world of gut health, don't worry. We'll start with the basics, like the fact that your digestive system—but most important, your intestines, which are a little farther down in the digestive tract than your stomach—is home to upward of 100 trillion beneficial microbes. A trillion is a hard number to conceptualize for most of us, so a helpful way to wrap your head around it is to think of it as one million *million* bacteria. One trillion dollar bills laid next to each other would extend from the earth to the sun and back with many miles left to spare. Do that a hundred times and you start to get at least a rough idea of what's living inside of you, in your vast gut garden. There are so many bacteria in your gut that you actually have upward of ten times more bacteria in your gastrointestinal system than you have human cells in your body. You could say you are a sophisticated, beautiful host for the microbiome metropolis.

Together, all these bacteria make up your gut microbiome, which is a vast gut garden that includes not just bacteria but also fungi, viruses, and parasites. You and your gut bacteria have evolved over millennia as symbiotic organisms, which means your body provides them with certain things they need to thrive—for example, a place to live and food to eat—and in exchange, they perform vital functions for you—for example, helping you digest food or protecting you from pathogenic bacteria or viruses that threaten to make you sick.

Together, all these microbes create an ecosystem, a whole little world inside your gut. This highly sophisticated microbiome metropolis is where a lot of important bodily processes originate or occur. We often focus on digestion when we talk about the gut and the microbiome, but your gut bacteria play a role in way more than just digestion. The microbiome is intricately connected to your metabolism, hormone, brain, and immune function. Your gut is also intricately connected to your mental and emotional health. Your gut is where 95 percent of the serotonin and 50 percent of the dopamine (your main "feel-good" neurotransmitters) in your body are made and kept. The microbiome exercises unbelievable control over your mood and nervous system as in these examples:

* An increase in certain types of gut bacteria has been directly connected to anxiety and depression.
* The development of PTSD has been linked to changes in the gut bacteria after a traumatic event.
* An increase in certain types of gram-negative bacteria in the gut at the end of the menstrual cycle is associated with premenstrual symptoms like anxiety, irritability, and food cravings.

Weighing about five pounds, these bacteria wield a lot of power over your mood and behavior. In another example, emerging research is showing that our gut bacteria can actually tell us what to eat and influence our mental health until we do their bidding. Researchers have shown that introducing certain types of bacteria into the microbiomes of animals can completely change their behavior when it comes to food choices. How does this work? The most likely explanation is that metabolites produced by bacteria carry information from the gut to the brain, telling the host whether it needs a particular kind of food. If you've ever tried to cut out sugar, you've likely seen this mechanism in action. When we eat a lot of sugar, sugar-eating bacteria are allowed to overgrow in number, feeding off the sugar we consume. When we try to reduce the amount of sugar in our diet, these bacteria panic at the loss of food. In an effort to save themselves, they attempt to get us to eat sugar again by changing our taste buds and influencing our opioid and cannabinoid receptors as well as neurotransmitters like dopamine and serotonin. This is why we experience intense sugar cravings and often feel anxious, cranky, and tired when we start a sugar detox. As you can see, we shouldn't underestimate the power of the microbiome.

What's Up with Your Gut?

As I mentioned earlier, there's a whole little world living inside your gut, and it has a massive influence on your entire body's health. When something's wrong with your gut, you'll likely feel it in your mood, metabolism, immune system, and so much more. But what disrupts a healthy gut in the first place? Here are five common gut health issues I see all the time in my practice.

1. **Bacterial Dysbiosis.** As we just learned, your microbiome contains a delicate balance of microbial species that live in harmony with you. Unfortunately, factors like medication overuse (particularly antibiotics, which can wipe out populations of good bacteria as well as kill bad ones), stress, and poor-quality foods can disrupt this essential balance of bacteria. As a result, "bad" bugs can start to replicate and grow, crowding out beneficial probiotic bacteria. This is called *bacterial dysbiosis*, which essentially means "an imbalance of gut bacteria."

2. **Leaky Gut.** Ahh, *leaky gut*. Such a cute term, isn't it? In a healthy gut, the intestinal lining—which is where the nutrients from the foods you eat get absorbed into the bloodstream through the lining—contains structures called *tight junctions*. These tight junctions act as tiny bouncers, regulating what's allowed to pass from the digestive tract to the inside of the body. When leaky gut occurs, the intestinal lining becomes damaged, and these tight junctions get a little less . . . well . . . tight. As a result, things that shouldn't penetrate the intestinal lining (like food particles, bad bacteria, and toxins) start to slip through into the bloodstream. As you can probably guess, this loss of control over what stays out and what gets in can wreak havoc in the area and cause chronic systemic inflammation that sabotages your health.

3. **Small Intestinal Bacterial Overgrowth.** Mostly referred to as SIBO, this increasingly common condition can lead to a wide variety of digestive problems such as irritable bowel syndrome (IBS), bloating, histamine intolerance, and acid reflux. SIBO is also associated with mental health issues like anxiety and brain fog. It happens when bacteria in the large intestines overgrow into the small intestines. So how does SIBO happen? Your gut is composed of the small and the large intestines, and when you're not eating, you have something called the *migrating motor complex* (MMC), which is supposed to push gut bacteria down into the large intestine, where most of them live. When this process isn't working as well as it should, bacteria that are meant to migrate down, instead grow up into the small intestine, where they don't belong.

4. **Candida Overgrowth.** The word *candida* refers to the *Candida albicans* fungus, which is the most common yeast in the human gastrointestinal system. Ideally, candida occurs in small amounts in all our digestive tracts as part of an overall healthy mycobiome balance (the prefix *myco* denoting the fungal species of the larger microbiome). Sometimes, however, things can get knocked out of balance—often when there is a decrease in beneficial bacteria, such as with a course of antibiotics or a diet high in sugar—and this allows candida to grow out of control. This not only causes the symptoms of candida overgrowth to occur, but also creates a situation where other opportunistic bacteria, yeasts, and parasites can take over and wreak havoc on your physical and mental health.

5. **Food Sensitivities.** Number five on the list of common gut health issues I see in my telehealth clinic is food sensitivities. Both a cause and a consequence of leaky gut, food intolerances and sensitivities are becoming more common with each passing year. Like seasonal allergies, food sensitivities are immune-mediated—

but they can oftentimes result in a more delayed reaction than a sneezing fit after hanging out with your friend's cat or dog. Sensitivities are complicated because you may be able to digest certain amounts of foods you are sensitive to without an issue, but eating that food every day may gradually affect your health in surprising ways, such as causing anxiety or triggering rashes. These symptoms don't often occur immediately after eating but instead hours or even days later.

The microbiota are one of the main regulators of the gut-feeling connection, which is why so much of the Gut-Feeling Plan and the dietary suggestions in chapter 5 are centered around supporting a healthy gut microbiome. That said, it's not the only fascinating way these two aspects of your health are connected. Your gut has its own nervous system that is playing a role in your gut-feeling interactions, too.

The Gut and the Nervous System

Earlier we talked about butterflies and stomach grumbles as evidence of the gut-feeling connection, but of course this phenomenon goes far deeper than these small moments in time. The gut and the brain are intricately connected largely by one facet of the nervous system, called the *enteric nervous system*. The enteric nervous system (ENS) is a division of the peripheral nervous system that actually *lives within the walls of the gastrointestinal tract*. There are some 200 to 600 million neurons of the ENS embedded in the mucosal lining and muscles that make up the gut; these are found from the very start of the digestive tract (the mouth) to the very end (the colon).[1] The ENS works directly with the central nervous system to modulate digestion—mainly processes like initiating swallowing and the release of digestive enzymes that help you absorb your food—but it's also involved in other bodily processes, including the stress response. The ENS communicates directly with the central nervous system. In fact, the two systems send messages back and forth throughout your day and even when you sleep. That means that every time you feel a pang of anxiety or shame or happiness or excitement, your brain and gut are communicating and responding accordingly.

With this in mind, it's easy to see how emotional health can be such a big disrupter of digestive health. Think about it: Your nervous system can turn digestion on and off, influence your gut bacteria, and even affect gut motility at a moment's notice! When we talk about digestive issues, it's easy to put all the focus on food, but the existence of the enteric nervous system means that food is only part of the equation. So while I wholeheartedly believe that food can act as medicine or a trigger for disease, that's not where the conversation ends! If you've been eating healthy foods but you're still dealing with digestive issues, there's a great chance your stress levels—and the enteric nervous system—are playing a part. The research doesn't lie:

- Stress is known to increase intestinal permeability, leading to conditions like leaky gut.
- Stress increases your susceptibility to chronic inflammation in the colon and gastrointestinal (GI) tract.
- Stress is associated with gastrointestinal disease, including functional bowel disorders like SIBO, inflammatory bowel disease, peptic ulcer disease, and gastroesophageal reflux disease.
- Stress is a known trigger for flare-ups in inflammatory bowel disease like Crohn's disease and ulcerative colitis.

Being under chronic sustained stress can sabotage your digestion to the point that practically no matter what you eat, you're going to have trouble digesting it in a way that is comfortable and helps you absorb and utilize the nutrients in the food you eat. Why? Because of the almost endless connections between your brain and your gut, starting with the enteric nervous system.

The Nervous System—The Gears of the Gut-Feeling Connection

The enteric nervous system is one component of a larger branch of your nervous system called the *autonomic nervous system* (ANS). The ANS is a branch of the nervous system that influences internal organs and regulates involuntary physiological processes like heart rate, blood pressure, digestion, sexual arousal, respiration, and the fight-or-flight response. The ANS is divided into three branches—the sympathetic nervous system, the parasympathetic nervous system, and the enteric nervous system. Let's talk about the sympathetic nervous system—which is known for regulating the fight-or-flight response. The SNS is one of our body's most incredible systems, intricately designed to protect us from harm and give our bodies and brains the tools they need to escape danger and stay alive. When we encounter a stressor—for example, when a loud noise goes off near us or we almost get hit by a soccer ball at our kid's game—our body launches into sympathetic activation. In an instant, the amygdala (an almond-shaped part of the brain that regulates fear) sends a sort of SOS signal to the hypothalamus, which is kind of like a central command center for the fight-or-flight response.

Through a very complex web of communications, called the *hypothalamic-pituitary-adrenal axis* (HPA axis), this signal makes its way to the adrenal glands, which start producing adrenaline, leading to instant physiological changes that we're all familiar with. For example, our heart rate increases, our muscles tense, our breathing becomes shallower, glucose is released into our bloodstream, and our digestion slows down so we can direct blood and energy to other areas of the body. Your lungs even expand their capacity so you can get the most oxygen in the fewest possible breaths. All of this happens in an instant. You have that surge of adrenaline; your heart feels like ice and your brain goes totally haywire for a split second. You are ready to fight or flee. If the threat doesn't immediately pass, the HPA axis activates another series of communications to keep the sympathetic nervous system activated for more than just a few seconds. This leads to the release of cortisol—known as the body's main stress hormone—by the HPA axis.

Chronic overactivation of the autonomic nervous system, either through physiological stressors (such as chronic gut problems or chronic infections like mold toxicity or Lyme disease) or psychological stressors (such as chronic stress or trauma) or both can trigger something called *dysautonomia*. Dysautonomia is a dysfunction of the autonomic nervous system, particularly in that the parasympathetic response is decreased and the sympathetic response is on overdrive. Dysautonomia can be diagnosed on its own, but it is usually associated with other health problems such as chronic fatigue syndrome, chronic Lyme disease, chronic mold toxicity, or autoimmune conditions like multiple sclerosis (MS) and fibromyalgia. When a person has dysautonomia, their body is in many ways stuck in an overactivation of the sympathetic response, perpetually in a state of hypervigilance. The truth is, this is not just about dysautonomia. Dysautonomia is just one end of a larger dysregulated nervous system spectrum in which the stress response is constantly firing, and the body is unable to calm down and return to a safe, relaxed, restful state.

Physiological versus Psychological Stressors

As we're learning about the autonomic nervous system and the inner workings of the gut-feeling connection, I use simple examples of stressors—for example, getting hit by a soccer ball or hearing a loud noise. I find that this is the best way to understand how the nervous system works. But the truth is, we all know that stray soccer balls or loud noises aren't the only stressors we encounter. Most of us can admit that those quick moments of stress are the least of our worries. The stressors most of us struggle with daily are more chronic, more adult, and more modern. There are physical stressors, which I talk about a lot with my patients that include factors like these:

+ Poor nutrition and nutrient deficiencies
+ Underlying gut health issues
+ Exposure to toxins
+ Biotoxins like Lyme disease and mold toxicity
+ Lack of exercise

- Chronic pain
- Chronic disease
- Poor sleep

There are also psychological stressors, which we'll learn more about in the next chapter, that include factors like these:

- Chronic stress about work, finances, relationships, health, or any number of other factors
- Situational anxiety and depression
- Emotions like anger or shame
- Trauma and multigenerational trauma

Both physiological stressors and psychological stressors can send us into chronic sympathetic activation and a fight-or-flight state, contributing to health issues. These stressors are far more dangerous than the stray soccer ball or a loud noise as they're more difficult to recover from and changing them often requires time and effort. But you don't have to suffer endlessly. In upcoming chapters, we'll be diving into just how we can send the ANS back to a state of calm.

Rest and Digest: The Parasympathetic Nervous System and the Vagus Nerve

Regardless of how long a stressor lasts, the flip side of our nervous system, our parasympathetic nervous system (PNS), kicks in when the threat has passed and we feel safe again. Known as our rest-and-digest system, the PNS helps slow our heartbeat and brings us back to a state of peace and calm. These two components of the autonomic nervous system act as alternating levels, like the accelerator and the brake—when one gets activated, the other goes into the off position. Unfortunately, our stress-filled modern lives paired with this ancient system can mean that sometimes we get stuck in a chronic sympathetic activation. When we suffer from chronic sustained stress, our SNS is constantly activated, our adrenal glands are constantly pumping out cortisol and adrenaline, and our PNS rarely has a chance to kick in and help us wind down. This can cause something called *adrenal fatigue* or *HPA axis dysfunction*, which is when the stress response system starts to go haywire, causing you to produce stress hormones all the time. The good news is that you can actively support the parasympathetic nervous system with certain calming and soothing activities (think: spending time in nature; playing with a puppy; taking long, deep breaths; or reading a good book).

Parasympathetic activation is something that I work with on an almost hourly basis with patients, and there's a long list of practices and tips to get out of autonomic dysfunction. Restoring parasympathetic response and getting out of chronic sympathetic overactivation are at the heart of the Gut-Feeling Plan. Why? Because along with supporting gut health through proper nutrition, these are the best tools we have to reduce the burden of negative emotions on the body and our health. All the practices for activating the PNS involve something called the *vagus nerve,* an incredible nerve that travels from the base of your brain down your body and into your abdomen. The vagus nerve is like the lever we use to get our body out of an SNS response and back into a state of rest and digestion. If the parasympathetic nervous system is a machine we have to turn on to restore a healthy gut-feeling connection, the vagus nerve is the switch itself.

The vagus nerve explains how, exactly, the gut and brain send messages to each other so specifically and immediately throughout the day and night. The vagus nerve is the longest nerve in the body—the word *vagus* literally means "winding" or "wandering"—and it travels from the base of the brain into almost every major organ, including the digestive system and the heart. Your vagus nerve is the most important nerve in your parasympathetic (rest, digest, and repair) nervous system. The vagus nerve explains how emotions can "trigger" physiological changes in your body so immediately and why emotions seem to affect far corners of the body in ways that are hard to explain or articulate. The vagus nerve is essentially the main component of the PNS and has a massive influence on the body's functioning, including the mood and the heart rate. If we want to get out of chronic sympathetic activation, we have to target the vagus nerve. Why? Because in many ways, the vagus nerve is the modulator of the gut-feeling connection. For example, the authors of one study explain that patients with IBS are more likely to have low vagus nerve activity.[2] Not to mention, nerve endings of the vagus nerve in the gut have 5-HT receptors, which work to sense serotonin secreted by gut bacteria and send signals to the brain that release antianxiety chemicals there.

We've made big strides in research concerning the vagus nerve in recent years, but the truth is that theories surrounding the importance of the vagus nerve have been floating around for centuries. In 1872, Darwin himself even acknowledged that there was a fascinating connection between the heart and the brain. In one of his early publications, he wrote that "when the heart is affected it reacts on the brain; and the state of the brain again reacts through the pneumo-gastric [vagus] nerve on the heart; so that under any excitement there will be much mutual action and reaction between these, the two most important organs of the body."[3]

So how do we know how healthy our vagus nerve is? Vagal nerve activity is often described as *vagal tone*. Having a low vagal tone—meaning less activity of the vagus nerve—can be connected to a wide range of health issues and imbalances. For example, poor or low vagal tone is associated with these issues:

- Depression
- Chronic inflammation and immune dysregulation
- Anxiety
- General sensitivity to stress
- Emotional reactivity and poor inhibitory control
- Digestive problems like slow GI motility, constipation, IBS, low stomach acid or hypochlorhydria, and poor absorption of nutrients like vitamin B12
- Poor blood sugar control
- Poor heart rate variability (HRV)
- High resting heart rate
- Chronic fatigue
- Difficulty calming down and meditating
- Higher blood pressure

But to sum things up in one sentence: Vagal tone makes you vulnerable both to physical and psychological stressors.

The Endocannabinoid System and the Gut-Feeling Connection

I know we've covered a lot of bodily systems so far in this chapter, but there's another major system of your body, one that is intricately involved in your gut-feeling connection, that you should know about. This system is called the *endocannabinoid system (ECS)*, and it exists as a massive network of receptors, enzymes, and compounds that the body naturally produces, called *endocannabinoids*. These compounds are eerily similar to certain compounds found in the cannabis plant, called *CBD* and *THC*. The ECS plays a surprisingly large role in our mood, stress response, and gut health. In fact, it's often described as the body's master regulatory system. It has already been linked to a wide range of health factors—such as the stress response and the digestive system—and is involved in an equally wide range of disorders, anything from autism and migraines to fibromyalgia or irritable bowel syndrome.[4,5] Scientists are now able to measure endocannabinoid "tone" much like vagal tone to determine the health of this system. There's still a lot we don't know about the ECS, but we do know it is involved in the larger picture of the gut-feeling connection. The good news is that it appears that many of the lifestyle practices and therapies that benefit our gut and nervous system, such as mindfulness and proper nutrition, can positively influence the ECS. I won't delve too deeply into the ECS here, but know that it's an integral part of the gut-feeling connection and that you're bringing balance to this bodily system as well throughout the Gut-Feeling Plan. For now, it's worth having this system on your radar.

I know the sections above got pretty granular, so let's recap what we learned:

- First, the gut is the center of it all. Our microbiome contains trillions of bacteria with an innate intelligence that affects not only our body but our mind.
- The gut has its own nervous system, called the *enteric nervous system,* which is part of a larger branch of the nervous system called the *autonomic nervous system.*
- The main branches of the ANS are the parasympathetic nervous system (rest-and-digest nervous system) and the sympathetic nervous system, which is our fight-or-flight response.
- The vagus nerve, a long winding nerve that travels from the brain to the gut, is the main connector between the gut and brain.

I know all these systems can seem overwhelming and complicated. How can you make sure all these parts of your body are functioning in harmony? The good news is that restoring balance to the microbiome, strengthening the vagus nerve, and flipping the on switch of the PNS is not nearly as complicated as you might think. Small daily practices can easily make a difference. For example, a simple meditation practice can get you out of fight or flight, and probiotics can modulate the gut microbiome, supporting the bacteria that can improve symptoms of anxiety and depression.

That said, the main foundation of a healthy gut-feeling connection is nutrition. The foods we eat have an undeniable effect on our microbiome, nervous system, and gut-feeling connection.

Food as the Foundation of the Gut-Brain Connection

The wellness world has no shortage of food fights, but the biggest one of them all is between the diet culture and the anti-diet culture. On one side, the diet culture implies that you aren't good enough unless you perpetually are on a strict diet and work out obsessively. The diet culture will rarely say it out loud, but the message is resoundingly clear: Shame and obsess your way to weight loss and health. On the other side, you have the anti-diet culture. As well intentioned as it may be, it can become another form of dysfunctional tribalism, and in the name of body positivity, fall into the trap of suspending health logic and pushing solutions that might not work for everyone.

Unfortunately, both sides often result with a person feeling unwell, shamed, and stressed. The solution to toxic diet culture tribalism is not to swing from one extreme to the other.

Many of the patients who come to me have been suffering every single day for years, and oftentimes some of that pain and suffering can be tied back to certain foods that do not agree with their physiology and contribute to their health problems. Also, certain foods do not agree with *anyone's* physiology because they are processed manufactured foods that have no nutritional value but a lot of potential to do harm. We shouldn't normalize restriction or dieting for the sake of dieting, but neither should we normalize foods that, based on extensive scientific research, have the potential to sabotage our physical and mental health in the name of body positivity. I try to focus on what will help my patients suffer less, so they can be their happiest selves both physically and mentally. It's not unhealthy or toxic to want to feel great and have a basic awareness that some foods can raise inflammation, mess up your blood sugar, hurt your digestion, and make you feel fatigued, anxious, or down. By the same token, don't let an upside-down culture sell you shame disguised as a wellness practice. Remember, you can't heal a body you hate. You can't shame your way to wellness, and you can't obsess your way to health.

Let's end the tired food wars, the battle of diet culture versus anti-diet culture. Let's end this binary reductive thinking and find food peace, the third way.

The beauty of functional medicine is bio-individuality. We are all different, with different experiences, preferences, and paths. Healing is a beautiful spectrum of light and color, emanating outward in a million different ways.

Every bite of food we put in our mouths contains messages to our body that promote either health and vitality or disease and distress. Food plays a fundamental role in the health of your body, from your immune system and metabolism to your hormone health and heart health. Virtually no part of your body is unaffected by your nutrition—from your liver to your hair, skin, and nails to the health of your eyes. Obvious strong connections can be drawn between what you eat and how you feel on a daily basis.

The gut-feeling connection is certainly no exception. The foods we eat are fundamental to the health of our gut and our brain. The nutrients we eat are what the bacteria in our gut feed on and what determines whether the beneficial bacteria in our guts struggle or flourish. As we've already learned, these bacteria have a huge influence on our brain—they communicate directly with our brain by producing neurotransmitters like dopamine and serotonin, which largely regulate our mood and emotions.

In later chapters, we'll be diving into all the foods that are foundational to a healthy gut and brain. But at this moment, I want to call out a handful of foods that are well known for sabotaging the gut and brain and, in turn, our mental health.

Don't panic! I don't expect you to never eat any of the foods below again. Part of achieving optimal health is recognizing that the human body is incredibly resilient and that it can handle a certain amount of stress, including physiological stressors from less-than-optimal foods. Nobody's perfect, and we're all human—and our bodies are designed to protect us and help us thrive, even in the face of challenges. So instead of playing the blame game with the foods below, I challenge you to instead just reflect on the role the following five foods play in your life. Ask yourself:

- How often are you consuming these foods?
- How do you feel before and after?
- Do you have a hunch that any of these foods affect your gut or brain negatively?
- Is there space in your life to have more awareness and intention around those foods?

In the Gut-Feeling Plan, we'll talk about some of these foods again, but I won't ask you to remove them completely. Why? Because this book isn't about food sensitivities or elimination diets—it's about achieving health and joy through nutrition, lifestyle, and self-compassion and acceptance. Throughout the 21-Day Gut-Feeling Plan, I'll ask you to observe yourself and your habits and ask yourself: *Is this feeding my gut and my brain? What about my head and my heart?* Keep that in mind as you move through the following section. What I find is that, with a little bit of education and self-awareness, we naturally start to shift our lifestyles without any real effort at all.

1. Sugar

For years we've known that sugar is one of the main contributing factors to the obesity epidemic. But the truth is, the negative consequences of too much sugar go far beyond our waistlines. As someone who studies nutrition and sees patients every single day, I can say that sugar is at the top of the list of dietary factors sabotaging our health as humans. Sugar is connected not only to diabetes and obesity—which many of us already know—but also to heart disease, dementia, autoimmune diseases, and essentially every other leading cause of disability and death in the world. I don't mean to scare you, but the truth is that the sugar problem is big.

On an average day, American adults aged twenty and older consume about 17 teaspoons of added sugar per day, which *adds up to about 60 pounds of sugar every year.* As you can guess, this has devastating consequences for our health and damages the gut and the brain. In fact, I'd go as far as to say that sugar hijacks our nervous system, our brains, and our gut microbiome. The sweet stuff is fuel for the anxiety fire. Many studies have shown that the more sugar you eat (specifically the refined kind), the worse your anxiety can be. And research has found that high levels of serotonin are making anxiety levels worse. And guess what also raises serotonin levels? Yep, you guessed correctly—sugar. And this can all be traced back to your microbiome. The correct balance of bacteria in your microbiome is responsible for how healthy you are. You can support healthy or unhealthy bacteria by the foods you choose to eat. Sugar is the perfect fuel for all types of bad bacteria, including yeast overgrowths such as candida. Studies have shown that lower levels of beneficial bacteria, specifically *Bifidobacterium longum* and *Lactobacillus helveticus*, are found in those struggling with anxiety.[6]

Then there's blood sugar. When you consume too much sugar, it can lead to blood sugar spikes, imbalances, and insulin resistance. When your blood sugar is on a roller coaster, it throws off your hypothalamic-pituitary-adrenal axis (HPA axis), which is responsible for releasing cortisol, your stress hormone. The fight-or-flight response that happens when you are stressed or anxious is due to an increased stream of cortisol. Because of the constant ups and downs, your body never really gets a chance to calm down, which further perpetuates the feelings of anxiety. It's been shown that diets mainly consisting of sugar and high-glucose foods raise anxiety, but switching to a low-sugar diet can drastically lower anxiety after just four weeks![7]

Sugar has a unique effect on our brain that causes our brain's reward system to light up. Immediately after eating sugar, we feel happier and even more relaxed thanks to the release of chemicals called *opioids* in our brain. This feels amazing in the moment, but just as is true with drugs or alcohol, these effects don't last long, and eventually we are left craving more sugar. If we don't get our regular sugar fix, we can end up with intense cravings, withdrawal symptoms, and bingeing.

Even sugar alternatives like sucralose and aspartame can sabotage your health. Multiple studies have shown that these sugar alternatives can exacerbate irritable bowel diseases like ulcerative colitis and Crohn's disease by promoting bad bacteria and gut inflammation. I wish I didn't have to deliver this news—I know how much some of you love your diet soda—but I'll never sell you short by (fake) sugarcoating the truth.

You're a human moving through this world, and my guess is that you already have a sense that sugar is affecting your gut and brain in a negative way, so let's move on to our next common offender: alcohol.

2. Alcohol

I know I will lose some friends here, but among my patients, I see unhealthy relationships with alcohol all too often when it comes to a healthy gut and brain. The reality is alcohol is a neurotoxin that ruins millions of lives every single year. The normalization and glamorization of drinking creates more problems in people's health and the health of their relationships. As with most things, it exists on a spectrum. Alcohol isn't an effective coping mechanism for stress, anxiety, and loneliness; for most people, I'd argue that it just takes those issues and magnifies them.

I have seen countless people who get anxious and panicky when they lack access to alcohol. Others have entire friendships and social circles centered around alcohol. Without alcohol, we find it much more difficult to numb and distract ourselves, check out, or lubricate our worries and emotions.

Alcohol is a super saboteur of the gut-feeling connection. For one, it leads to microbiome issues and exacerbation of leaky gut. One study showed that it can increase intestinal permeability and cause inflammation in other organs, including the brain. Another study published in *Scientific Reports* showed that people who drank a few times a week had lower total brain volume in early middle age (people from thirty-nine to forty-five years old).[8] This is associated with brain fog, poor memory, mood changes, and other neurological symptoms. Alcohol is often used to curb anxiety, but that is far from a good idea. Research has shown that alcohol consumption is associated with a worsening of anxiety disorders over time. Studies have also shown that drinking alcohol can rewire the brain and contribute to feelings of anxiety.[9]

Alcohol can also trigger inflammation that affects your entire body—and that includes the brain. In fact, the brain might be particularly at risk, since an overload of inflammation can trigger an inflammatory autoimmune response against your brain and nervous system. The consequences of this are often an erratic mood, negative emotions, and feelings of anxiety and depression. Inflammation can also damage your blood-brain barrier (BBB), which can lead to something called *leaky brain* and *oxidative stress* in the hypothalamus, which is the part of the brain responsible for regulating appetite and weight, body temperature, emotions, behavior, memory, growth, salt and water balance, sex drive, and sleep-wake cycle (is that all?). Needless to say, the consequences of this, which include brain fog, concentration, and attention issues, are something you want to avoid.

The truth is, most of us already know these facts about alcohol just based on our own experiences. I don't know a single person who hasn't had at least one negative experience with alcohol. Alcohol may make us feel carefree, connected, and confident in the moment, but most of us know the uncomfortable anxiety of waking up after a night of drinking. By damaging your gut and affecting your brain, alcohol consumption, especially binge drinking, is one of the easiest ways to sabotage your mental and physical health. One study that observed people who participated in Dry January showcases this fact extremely well.[10] After just a month of no booze:

- 71 percent slept better.
- 67 percent had more energy.
- 58 percent lost weight.

- 57 percent had better concentration.
- 54 percent had better skin.

When we stop consistently giving our brains neurotoxins, our brains have a powerful capacity for healing. Now, you already know that I'm not making any hard-and-fast rules for the 21-Day Gut-Feeling Plan, but my recommendation is always to limit alcohol to special occasions and to keep it to small amounts of low-alcohol, low-sugar, organic, biodynamic wine and hard kombucha.

3. Processed and Packaged Foods

I know lumping all processed and packaged foods into one category may seem extreme—there are so many different types; aren't some of them pretty healthy?—but I'm doing this here to make a specific point. Processed and packaged foods make up a giant category that includes essentially anything that isn't fresh and in its original state. Most things in the middle aisles of the grocery store are packaged and processed, while anything in the produce and meat aisle is typically unprocessed. Most processed foods and packaged foods lack the essential nutrient that gut bacteria need to flourish: fiber. Fiber, especially prebiotic fiber, is the food your bacteria eat. You can think of fiber as a type of fertilizer for your good gut bacteria—you know, the ones that help regulate the nervous system and produce neurotransmitters. This type of dietary fiber is digested more slowly by your body and acts as a source of food for your gut's healthy bacteria so they can multiply. When you eat foods rich in prebiotics, you are providing just the right kind of fuel your gut needs to thrive. It's not enough to eat only probiotics or prebiotics—your gut needs a healthy balance of both in order to keep your microbiome balanced.

Prebiotics are found in many fruits and vegetables, especially those that contain complex carbohydrates, such as fiber and resistant starch:

- Garlic
- Apples/apple cider vinegar
- Chicory root
- Jerusalem artichokes
- Bananas
- Dandelion root
- Oats
- Mangoes
- Berries
- Legumes
- Onions
- Potatoes
- Guava
- Leeks
- Oranges
- Asparagus
- Rice

Highly processed foods, which are generally low in fiber and prebiotic fiber, are associated with bad gut microbes linked to poorer health markers. For example, one study published in the *International Journal of Environmental Research and Public Health* showed that participants who consumed less than three sources of fruits and vegetables daily had 24 percent higher odds of a diagnosis of anxiety disorder.[11]

In a practical sense, when we rely on processed and packaged foods, there's just less room in our diet for fresh fruits and vegetables, nuts and seeds, and other ingredients that provide us with beneficial fiber, vitamins, and minerals that we need to thrive. This can create its own set of problems, since studies have shown that those who eat a diet rich in minimally processed foods like vegetables, nuts, eggs, and seafood are more likely to harbor beneficial gut bacteria and have better mental and physical health. For example, one study on adults with depression showed that working with a dietician for twelve weeks to make adjustments, such as eating less junk food and eating more foods richer in nutrients (such as produce, fish, fruit, and vegetables) led to almost a third of the participants achieving remission from their depression.[12]

The problem with processed foods, and the reason they've become such a big part of our diet, is the fact that they are just so darn convenient, fast, and cheap. We've created a world where it's easier to pick these foods than the ones that fuel our gut and our brain. Eating nutrient-deficient foods has become so ubiquitous that eating like humans would have eaten for thousands of years is now labeled as "restrictive," "radical," or "toxic diet culture."

Tackling the problem of sugar, alcohol, and processed foods may seem insurmountable; after all, they're all pretty big parts of our society. The good news is that studies show that just a few days after you swap out nutrient-deficient foods for nutrient-dense foods, the makeup of your gut microbiome starts to shift and improve pretty quickly. This is true not just in the actual makeup of the bacteria themselves, but also in the genes they express. One study found that positive changes can begin to happen in hours as opposed to days or weeks.[13] Knowing this, just imagine what you can do in 21 days!

CHAPTER 3

Feelings

Stress, Trauma, and
How Shameflammation Finds Its Home

Throughout my years as a functional medicine practitioner, I've spent innumerable days educating people on the concept of food as medicine, teaching them about the pitfalls of nutrient-poor junk foods. My goal has always been to make my patients and readers aware of the link between what they eat and how they feel—a connection that conventional medicine tends to either underestimate or ignore completely. I've helped hundreds of patients transform their health with this approach. From autoimmune diseases to chronic headaches to seasonal allergies to metabolic problems to IBS, virtually every single health condition in the world can be improved by proper nutrition.

With that said, the truth is that low-quality, inflammatory *junk foods aren't the only thing sabotaging our wellness.* In fact, many of us experience emotional factors that are just as damaging as any refined flour or high-fructose corn syrup. These emotional factors can take many forms, but some of the most common ones I see are chronic stress, toxic productivity, perfectionism, and trauma. When these negative emotional experiences are shoved away and ignored, it starts to show up in our physical body—in other words, we start to get Shameflammation.

In order to tame Shameflammation, we have to stop our emotional world from hurting our physical one. And to do that, we have to understand the ins and outs of how Shameflammation starts to build up in the first place. The perfect place to start is with the most universally experienced negative emotional experience—chronic stress.

Chronic Stress: The Ultimate Junk Food for the Body

The idea that stress is the worst junk food might seem somewhat out there. Could it possibly be worse than fast food or even soda? Researchers have been studying stress for years, and the consensus is that it's one of the single biggest factors in disease and illness. We're diving into stress first because most of us are already comfortable with the fact that we have stress in our lives, that it's probably affecting our health, and that we'd like to change that.

Stress not only makes us feel bad in the moment but also contributes to virtually every single health condition that exists. According to the American Psychological Association, chronic stress is directly linked to the six leading causes of death—heart disease, cancer, lung ailments, accidents, cirrhosis of the liver, and suicide.[1] Research has shown that more than 60 to 90 percent of doctor's visits are for stress-related ailments and complaints.[2] One study showed that healthcare expenditures are nearly 50 percent greater for people who report higher levels of stress, which makes sense when you realize that stress contributes to nearly all the health woes and aches and pains that we experience.[3] I'm talking about headaches, asthma and allergies, depression and anxiety, chronic muscle tension, acne, poor thyroid function, weight gain, indigestion, arthritis, blood sugar imbalance, decreased bone density and muscle tissue, nausea, yeast and urinary tract infections, and even colds and sinus infections. The list goes on and on. The truth is that you'd be hard-pressed to find a disease or illness that isn't made worse by higher levels of stress.

Here are just a few examples of how stress can affect our health in the long term:

• Stress triggers a chain reaction in your brain, as your hypothalamus sends orders to your adrenal glands to release cortisol and adrenaline, which can cause long-term changes in the structure and function of the brain that can contribute to mental health issues like insomnia.[4]

- Research shows that chronic stress alone can slow your metabolism, can sabotage your hunger signals, and can increase cravings enough to make you gain as much as 11 pounds every year.[5]
- Stress decreases the conversion of thyroid hormones T4 to T3, which can lead to low T3 syndrome and trigger autoimmune thyroid issues.[6]
- In the case of Alzheimer's, studies have shown that stress can drive the progression of the disease and exacerbate symptoms—and the symptoms of Alzheimer's impair one's quality of life, which creates more stress. In other words, stress begets stress, which begets stress, and so on.[7]
- Stress is known to increase intestinal permeability, leading to conditions like leaky gut, and to increase your susceptibility to chronic inflammation in the colon and GI tract.
- Stress is also connected to gastrointestinal disease, including functional bowel disorders, inflammatory bowel disease, peptic ulcer disease, and gastroesophageal reflux disease, and it is a known trigger for flare-ups in inflammatory bowel diseases such as Crohn's disease and ulcerative colitis.

Research shows that stress can even cause lasting changes in your body by changing your DNA. One study showed that chronic sympathetic activation, when left unchecked for too long, can eventually start to change the activity of a person's immune cells.[8] The study showed that chronic stress consistently triggered immune cells that are meant to fight infection, but no infection was actually present. This can lead to chronic inflammation, which is the root commonality of almost all diseases.

The Pressure of Perfectionism

Nowhere is perfectionism more dangerous than in the world of health and wellness. As I said at the very beginning of this book, I know many of us would love to be handed a list of items that would guarantee a life free of health issues. So would I! Many who are naturally drawn to wellness are also drawn to this idea that if they just do enough, if they just check everything off that list, they won't have to face uncertainty or suffering. Unfortunately, and I really hate to break this to you, no such list exists—and that's because no such human body exists! The human body is not capable of perfection, and therefore perfectionism is a guarantee of suffering and unhappiness.

By chasing an idea that we will be healthy and happy from morning to night all the days of our lives, we're setting ourselves up for certain failure. We can't possibly maintain a "perfect" diet and lifestyle. We can't eliminate junk food for life, sleep a blissful 8.5 hours every night, exercise every single day of our lives, or avoid all chemicals and toxins. Sometimes we will be tired, sick, or sad; our bodies will change and resist and rebel in big and small ways. We'll eat too much movie theater popcorn, we'll abandon our exercise routines for a few days or a few weeks or a few months, or we'll experience loss. We'll tear a muscle, have diarrhea, get a cold sore, or be diagnosed with an autoimmune disease, a blood sugar problem, or cancer.

Unfortunately, the images we see on social media and on television don't always reflect this reality. Instead, what we typically see is perfectly fit (and filtered), perfectly tanned bodies and smiling faces, which can leave us wondering what's wrong with us. When things go wrong with our bodies or our health, as they inevitably do, we are tempted to label ourselves as failures or berate ourselves for not doing enough. Unfortunately, this will only add to the already heavy burden of stress and negative emotions and can become a big contributor to Shameflammation. When we don't allow ourselves some space for imperfection, we really throw gasoline on the fire of Shameflammation.

All of this is why I decided to write this book and design the 21-Day Gut-Feeling Plan. In this plan, we throw perfectionism to the winds and allow ourselves to be radically, beautifully human. The goal of this book is to show you the path to be more "human being" and less "human doing." This book is about the lost art of slowing down, getting present, finding stillness, and listening to our gut feelings, which never lead us astray—the art of being well.

The Problem with Toxic Productivity

Many of us are always on the go. If not physically, at least mentally and emotionally, we are perpetually on. Of course you can't always control your packed schedule, and many of us are quick to feel left out, thinking we should be doing something fun, exciting, and novel at all hours of the day and night. With social media making it incredibly easy to post only the most carefully curated version of our lives, it's no surprise that seeing everyone's highlight reel makes us feel like we're constantly missing out on something bigger, better, and more fun. I have seen firsthand how much stress and anxiety FOMO (fear of missing out) can cause and how that heightened stress response can trigger health issues. You see, during periods of stress in your life, your body's stress hormone, cortisol, is on high alert. Even though this is a normal response, chronically high cortisol levels are not and may lead to a whole slew of health problems.

Our go-go-go lifestyle can also leave us little time to take care of ourselves. Chances are, the busier we are, the more likely we are to grab whatever is easiest and quickest to eat. Between work, social events, volunteering, and family activities, we have little time to prepare meals. This high-intensity lifestyle can also leave us sleepwalking through life, never quite expanding past our comfort zone or learning something new. How many times have you said to yourself, "I'd love to learn how to . . ." or "I've always wanted to try . . ." only to look back months (if not years) later, to realize you've never actually learned or tried that thing you're passionate about because of your packed schedule?

Times of stillness and reflection are absolutely key for emotional health, too. Having downtime gives us a chance to reflect on what is going on in the present moment. With a more mindful outlook on life, you can take the time necessary to unpack anything from your past—good or bad—and use it to make the best decisions for your future. Embracing some peace, quiet, and stillness is one of the best ways to calm stress and anxiety. With all the noise online and inside our minds, it is imperative to create spaces of stillness both within and without.

Clearly stress, including that caused by perfectionism and toxic productivity, often affects our ability to prevent illness or fend off disease, and it greatly damages our mental and physical resilience. But negative emotional experiences don't begin and end with stress—not even close. They also extend to other experiences, ones that are less universal and—let's be honest—less comfortable to talk about. These experiences involve more than checking off the items on our long to-do lists, being stuck in traffic, or getting through the busy season at work. They are about what's going on in our hearts and minds at the deepest level, right at their ooey-gooey core—sadness, trauma, grief, loneliness, jealousy, low self-esteem, anger, guilt, and shame. Oof, right? Just reading some of those words can knock the wind out of a person.

Your Deeper Feelings and Your Health

Let's dive straight in. Because as it turns out, you can pretty easily draw connections between different emotional experiences and your health. In one powerful example, there's broken heart syndrome, or stress cardiomyopathy. Research has shown that the risk of having a heart attack increases *21-fold* in the twenty-four hours after losing a loved one: As study researcher Elizabeth Mostofsky, a postdoctoral fellow in cardiovascular epidemiology, once explained to the *Boston Business Journal*: "Bereavement and grief are associated with increased feelings of depression, anxiety and anger, and those have been shown to be associated with increases in heart rate and blood pressure, and changes in the blood that make it more likely to clot, all of which can lead to a heart attack."[9,10]

Anger is another emotion that can have a powerful influence over our health. Unresolved or unmanaged anger has been linked to a wide range of health problems, including headaches, digestion problems, insomnia, high blood pressure, skin problems such as eczema, and heart attack and stroke. In one study published in the *Journal of Medicine and Life*, the authors write that "Anger can have a direct impact upon cardiovascular diseases through the HPA axis (brain-adrenal communication) and the sympathetic nervous system."[11] Another study showed that anger, hostility, and aggressiveness have been linked to the development of type 2 diabetes. For example, a study found individuals who scored the highest in the study's measurement of anger had a 34 percent increased risk of developing diabetes compared to those who scored the lowest.[12] It also revealed that anger contributed to unhealthy lifestyle behaviors, like smoking and high caloric intake, which ultimately led to obesity and eventually diabetes.

Another good example of the effects of emotion on our physical health is in the case of loneliness and isolation, which almost all of us have experienced at some point during the COVID-19 pandemic. Research has linked social isolation and loneliness to higher risks for a variety of physical and mental conditions: high blood pressure, heart disease, obesity, a weakened immune system, anxiety, depression, cognitive decline, Alzheimer's disease, and even death. In one final interesting example, researchers studied people with multiple sclerosis and found that low self-esteem was correlated with fatigue, suggesting that how the patients saw and valued themselves could influence their symptoms.[13]

Unresolved Past Trauma in Your Body

We often think of the gut-feeling connection as something that occurs only in the short term, or at least born of experiences from our lives as adults. But research has shown that it's not just current emotional experiences that affect our health; it's also the experiences we may have thought we'd left behind years ago. For example, it's well known that adverse childhood experiences (also known as ACEs) can increase your risk of developing physical health problems such as heart disease, obesity, diabetes, and cancer. In fact, child abuse and neglect is one of the biggest environmental causes of mental illness.[14] Another study, published in *Psychosomatic Medicine,* found that greater cumulative childhood stress—such as violence, parental separation, mental illness, divorce, or substance abuse—significantly increased the likelihood of being diagnosed with an autoimmune disease later in life.[15] Unresolved past trauma can lead to dysregulation of the autonomic nervous system and leave you on high alert all the time, stuck in that chronic fight-or-flight state. This can cause you to store that emotional distress in your body, where it eventually shows up as a physical health issue. This is the reason why my team and I cover these topics in every consultation with a new patient and integrate protocols to address this integral part of healing.

More recent trauma can also affect your health in myriad ways, and I'm 100 percent certain that all of us have experienced at least one trauma in our lives: the COVID-19 pandemic. It may have been traumatic for different reasons—maybe we lost a loved one, lost our business, or experienced loneliness and social isolation that is still affecting our mental health—but the result is the same for all of us: We experienced more sympathetic activation, and that can have lasting effects on our internal physiology and even our DNA expression.

Our DNA? you ask. We often think of stress and trauma as affecting our health only in the short term or in the form of pesky but not overly serious conditions like headaches or stomachaches, but the truth is, the effects of trauma can go much deeper than these everyday health woes. In fact, trauma can literally change the way your DNA expresses itself and can contribute directly to the development of disease. Your DNA serves as a sort of map for your body, telling it what to do and how to act on a cellular level. When your environment changes drastically, such as during a time of major stress or trauma, that DNA doesn't change fundamentally, but the way it's read by your body does change.

This area of research is called *epigenetics,* and it's the study of what genes get turned on and off by our lifestyle and environment. For example, you might have a gene for Alzheimer's or breast cancer, but depending on your lifestyle—for example, your low intake of alcohol or tobacco use—that gene may never get flicked on and, in turn, affect your life. Trauma and stress can be the difference between being diagnosed with a disease and not experiencing it. Interestingly, these epigenetic changes don't live and die with you.

A Word on Intergenerational Trauma

Trauma can be a single isolated instant, such as an accident or assault—in which case it's referred to as a *simple trauma*—but trauma can also be labeled complex if it occurs more than once or over a long period of time. One subset of complex trauma is called *intergenerational trauma,* which is also sometimes referred to as *transgenerational* or *multigenerational trauma.* This type of trauma is passed down through generations, from those who first experience a trauma to their descendants. What would have seemed like science fiction not too long ago has become a cutting-edge field in science. Many things get passed down through families, like genetic conditions and physical characteristics. In some cases, trauma can be inherited, too, like cellular heirlooms, woven deeply in the DNA. The symptoms of generational trauma may include hypervigilance, the sense of a shortened future, mistrust, aloofness, high anxiety, depression, panic attacks, nightmares, insomnia, a sensitive fight-or-flight response, and issues with self-esteem and self-confidence.

Generational trauma may lead to an overactive immune system, which can result in more autoimmune diseases or other inflammatory issues. Trauma also influences the microglia, the brain's immune system. When in a high trauma reactive state, the microglia eat away at nerve endings instead of enhancing growth and getting rid of damage. The microglia go haywire in the brain and cause depression, anxiety, and other brain problems. This can translate into genetic changes, which can be passed down to further generations. Research is being done concerning the generational trauma component to issues like metabolic syndrome, diabetes, weight gain, inflammatory cholesterol issues, autoimmune conditions, and brain health.

In one disturbing example, scientists studied the descendants of those who lived through what is known as the Holodomor, which was a human-made famine in Ukraine in the 1930s that resulted in the death of millions of people. The results of the study, which collected data from forty-four people from fifteen different Ukrainian families, showed that the coping mechanisms that the survivors adopted in the 1930s were clearly passed down through two and even three generations. Many of the participants

(continued)

had difficulty trusting people, anxiety about food scarcity, hoarding tendencies, low self-worth, social hostility, and risky health behaviors.[16] Some other research being conducted at the Icahn School of Medicine at Mount Sinai shows that the descendants of survivors of the Holocaust have distinctive stress hormone profiles. The data showed that those with intergenerational trauma have altered levels of circulating stress hormones. More specifically, they have lower levels of cortisol, a hormone that helps the nervous system and inflammation to calm down after a traumatic incident. This may predispose them to anxiety disorders and post-traumatic stress disorder.[17]

The good news? If trauma can be inherited, then healing can be, too. Healing yourself is healing your children's children and generations that you will never see. On a daily basis, I get to see my patients around the world breaking the ancestral chains of pain, shame, and health problems.

All this goes to show that our emotional world has a big impact on our physiology, a concept further explained by something called *polyvagal theory*.

Polyvagal Theory: How Shameflammation Finds Its Home in Your Nervous System

Earlier we learned about the vagus nerve and how it modulates the gut-feeling connection. Well, polyvagal theory helps us understand what it means to store stress and emotions in our body, and it helps us realize just how much uncontrolled negative emotional experiences can affect human physiology, especially that of the nervous and immune systems, in the long term. The polyvagal theory was proposed by a man named Stephen Porges, an expert on behavioral neuroscience. Before polyvagal theory was developed, we thought of stress as something that was finite—something that would turn on and then turn off a moment later. For example, you might hear a car alarm go off behind you and it would send your body into a temporary state of fight-or-flight response. But then once you realized it was just a car alarm, your body would immediately return to a state of relaxation, and all would be right in your internal world.

According to polyvagal theory, this is not quite so simple. Your nervous system isn't like a light switch that gets flicked on and off. Instead, there are a few possible states of the nervous system that someone could be in, including:

State 1. When the nervous system is in this state, we feel relaxed, at ease, and at peace. Think about a day spent hiking with friends, an amazing cup of tea on the porch with your partner, or the invigorated and peaceful feeling you get after making a new friend or connection. In the ventral-vagal social-engagement state, we have a clear head and heart and can connect and relate to other people around us and ourselves on a deep level. In this state, your body and mind feel in sync, your breathing is relaxed, and you feel like there's a direct unobstructed pathway between your head and heart. Ventral vagal social engagement is the antithesis of stress, negativity, and anxiety. As we move into the actionable portion of our journey, getting into this state will be our focus.

State 2. This is a nervous system state marked by acute stress (aka sympathetic activation). Think of it as how you feel when you're stuck in traffic, about to go into an interview, or on alert for a call from the doctor. In the sympathetic activation state, you are often plagued with jumpiness and racing thoughts, and you may experience muscle tension or an exacerbation of pain or chronic health issues. Unfortunately, many of us live in an almost constant state of sympathetic activation, which can make us always on the brink of anxiety or even a panic attack.

State 3. When your nervous system is in this state, you've struggled with sympathetic activation so much that your body shuts down and goes into a state similar to hibernation. You can think of this as a hole you can fall into, marked by fatigue, shame, sedation, anger, and depression. This dorsal vagal shutdown occurs when your body says, "No! I can't sustain this level of sympathetic activation anymore!" and it collapses. There's a good chance you've experienced this state at some point in your life, maybe after a particularly difficult time at work that left you totally burnt out, a breakup that left you emotionally spent, or a traumatic period in your life that made you feel like you needed to shut down to protect yourself.

Depending on which of these states you're in, the physiology of your body and the firing of the neurons in your brain will be different. These states change the way you perceive your entire reality, and the world starts to look either darker, scarier, and sadder or welcoming and peaceful. The same goes for your body—you will either feel at home and at peace in your body, or you will feel like it's more of a war zone that doesn't allow you to feel connected to yourself or the people around you.

Trauma, stress, and past experiences can change our nervous systems in ways that put us in a perpetual fight-or-flight state. I know many patients who feel chronically on edge, stuck with recurring negative thoughts and unable to pull themselves out of fight or flight and back to a state of calm and ease, where the gut-feeling connection can be one of mutual health and happiness. One of the things I love most about polyvagal theory is that it shows us it's not just our thoughts that control our psychological health—it's the way our nervous system has evolved to adapt to changing circumstances. So as much as I love practicing gratitude and thinking positive thoughts, I also know that if we want to really improve our overall health, we have to look closer at healing from the gut and the feeling side.

Autoimmunity and Your Relationship to Self

As I wrote in my book *The Inflammation Spectrum*, autoimmune disease is characterized by your body's loss of the ability to recognize what is its own tissue and what is an outside invader. As a result, your body starts attacking itself. All autoimmune diseases have this molecular mimicry process in common. The only difference between them is the area of the body that's being attacked. For example, in the case of Addison's disease, it's the adrenal glands; in Hashimoto's or Graves' disease, it's the thyroid; in ulcerative colitis or Crohn's disease, it's the digestive tract; in multiple sclerosis (MS), it's the brain and nervous system; and in rheumatoid arthritis, it's the joints. As you might already suspect, autoimmune diseases are intricately related to what goes on in the gut, which is the foundation of your immune system. For example, studies have shown that specific alterations in the gut microbial community can be linked to autoimmune conditions like lupus; researchers are even exploring microbiome-based treatments for patients.[18] Autoimmune skin conditions like psoriasis have been linked to decreased bacterial diversity in the gut and skin microbiome, too.[19]

If you go deep into the science of autoimmunity, on a physical level it is when the immune system has lost recognition of self and attacks itself. Think about that for a moment. By the time many of my patients have met me, they have spent years of their lives in varying degrees of feeling out of touch with their bodies and themselves. Day in and day out, they are mentally, emotionally, and spiritually attacking themselves and their body. What's going on in your gut is probably also what's going on in your head. The more stressed we are, the more we eat foods that don't align with our body, the more we self-criticize and shame ourselves, and the more we strive for perfection and not humanness. The further we get from following our intuition about what's healthiest for us, the more our internal physiology starts matching what's happening in our heads and hearts. As above, so below. As within, so without.

There is also research that shows challenging emotional experiences can be linked to autoimmune disease. For example, one study showed that those with post-traumatic stress disorder have a 60 percent increased risk of developing an autoimmune disease compared to those without a history of PTSD.[20] Scientists suspect the intense psychological stress of trauma causes physical changes that impact the immune system by creating chronic inflammation, activating genes, and accelerating immune cell production.[21]

If there's one piece of information that I hope you fully absorb by the time you're finished reading this book, it's that the physical and the psychological are not as separate as you think; and that if you don't take steps to improve the health and resilience of your body *and* your mind, you won't be able to achieve optimal health and happiness.

This type of trauma—indeed, all trauma—can massively influence people's health and well-being, but it can also influence their ability to create and maintain healthy lifestyle habits, such as making sound nutrition choices, exercising, and practicing self-care. A history of trauma increases the likelihood that you will drink too much, smoke, overeat, or remain sedentary. In recent years, we've gotten a lot more comfortable talking about trauma, mental health, and the parts of being human that have long been hidden away and ignored. That said, we still have a lot of progress to make, especially when it comes to the effects of trauma on physical health.

In his groundbreaking book *The Body Keeps the Score*, the author Bessel van der Kolk, MD, writes: "Traumatized people chronically feel unsafe inside their bodies: The past is alive in the form of gnawing interior discomfort." Dr. van der Kolk goes on: "Their bodies are constantly bombarded by visceral warning signs, and, to control these processes, they often become expert at ignoring their gut feelings and in numbing awareness of what is played out inside. They learn to hide from themselves." If you have a history of trauma, whether big or small, acute or intergenerational, my guess is that you can relate to that statement. I'll bet you know firsthand how trauma and physical health are intricately linked and you can relate to the concept of Shameflammation on a particularly deep level.

Now, I'm not going to tell you that this book or the 21-Day Gut-Feeling Plan will heal all of your trauma. Trauma is complex, it's big, and it requires a team of professionals working together to give you the best care possible. The point I'm trying to make is that when there is emotional suffering, there is almost always physical suffering. Your current and past emotional state don't exist just in your head; they can have a big effect on your body in the short and the long term. This book is the next step of your journey.

Barriers to Emotional Health: How Functional Medicine Can Help

If there's a strong emotional component to health and healing—which hopefully you agree with if you've read up until this point—then I think we can all agree it's important for us as a society to invest in ways to heal. It only makes sense that if the gut and brain are connected, if trauma can impact our health for generations, and if negative emotions and stress play a role in essentially every disease in the world, we'd want to create a healthcare system that knows how to support body and mind and the connection between the two. Unfortunately, we're far from achieving this goal. In fact, I'd go as far as to say that conventional medicine is quite bad at supporting us in this way. Instead, our Western healthcare system seems to throw gasoline directly on the fire of Shameflammation. As a result, not only do we have the problem of our emotional world sabotaging our physical one, but we also have the problem of there being substantial hurdles when we actually seek support.

I'd be surprised if you didn't already know that our world is failing in the area of mental health. Anyone that's ever tried to see a therapist likely understands how difficult it can be to get mental health support. Why? There are still so many barriers to high-quality affordable mental health services. One survey showed that 56 percent of 5,024 Americans surveyed want mental health services either for themselves or for a loved one, but about a third of them reported access issues, such as cost or poor insurance coverage, social stigma, lack of direction, and poor quality of care. The same survey showed that one in four people have to choose between getting mental health treatment and paying for daily necessities. Nearly one in five Americans noted they have had to choose between getting treatment for a physical condition and getting treatment for a mental health condition. Of those who can afford to get mental health support, about 38 percent must wait more than a week for treatments and 46 percent had to travel more than an hour round trip for an appointment.[22]

If it's hard to find an affordable mental health professional, it's even harder to find someone who is trained to draw connections between your *mental and physical health*. If you do try to bring up chronic stress or mental health in an appointment with a traditional medical doctor, they will most likely refer you to a psychologist or a psychiatrist. Conventional doctors are often not trained in psychology (at least not adequately), and psychologists are not always trained in physical health issues. Therefore, even if we can afford therapy, we end up being treated separately for mind and body by two different professionals who almost definitely don't know or talk to each other. Collaboration between the two is rare, so you end up trying to understand this mysterious connection between the physical and the emotional all on your own. This is a massive failure in our society, especially when you look at the statistics and realize that a shocking 60 percent of American adults have a chronic disease.

To put it simply, functional medicine is the thread that ties all the information in this book together. This subset of medicine gets serious about uncovering the root cause of health problems, focusing on lifestyle changes, nutrition, and mind-body therapies instead of simply covering up the symptoms with medication. It also teaches us to look at the body as one complex organism instead of separate unrelated parts. And most important, it teaches us that the gut-feeling connection is not only real but an integral part of overall health and happiness. The statistics don't lie. First-time functional medicine patient visits last anywhere from 60 to 120 minutes. Furthermore, compared to physicians practicing conventional medicine—who are suffering from burnout at devastating rates, as high as 50 percent according to some studies—about 43 percent of physicians practicing functional medicine plan to work into their seventies, indicating higher job satisfaction.[23]

Not surprisingly, functional medicine has its critics. Pejoratives like "quacks," "woo-woo," and "unscientific" are yelled from the sidelines.

But look at the statistics: A shocking 60 percent of American adults have a chronic disease, and 40 percent have two or more chronic diseases. Today someone will have a heart attack every 40 seconds, cancer is the second leading cause of death worldwide, 50 million Americans have an autoimmune disease, and almost half the population of the United States has either prediabetes or diabetes.[24]

As you already know, brain health problems are also on the rise. According to the CDC, around 20 percent of adults have a diagnosable mental disorder. Depression is now the leading cause of disability around the world. One in five American children ages three to seventeen (about 15 million kids) have a diagnosable mental, emotional, or behavioral disorder. Serious depression is worsening, especially among teens, with the suicide rate among teen girls reaching a forty-year high. The average young adult today has the same level of anxiety as the average psychiatric patient in the 1950s.[25] Anxiety impacts more than 40 million Americans, and Alzheimer's disease is the sixth leading cause of death in the United States. Since 1979, deaths due to brain disease have increased by 66 percent in men and a whopping 92 percent in women.

And despite all of this, the United States spends more on healthcare than the next ten top-spending countries combined. And even though we spend trillions of dollars, we rank last among all industrialized nations when it comes to living long, healthy lives. According to the *Journal of the American Medical Association* (*JAMA*), out of thirteen industrialized nations, the United States is the worst when it comes to years of life lost for adults and infant mortality rates.[26]

Most Americans take at least one medication a day. Prescription drugs now kill more people than heroin and cocaine combined. According to *JAMA*, more than 100,000 people die each year from the *proper* use of prescription drugs—not from overdosing or taking the wrong drug, but from the side effects of the "right drug."[27] Meanwhile, the drug industry is funding much of the scientific research we read today. Because of this conflict of interest, when it comes to chronic and autoimmune disease, mainstream medicine is trained to diagnose a disease and match it with a corresponding medication. This medicinal matching game leaves many frustrated when nothing changes with their health but a growing list of prescriptions to take.

In functional medicine, we're not anti-medication. We recognize that many people are alive because of these medications, and advancements in modern medicine have brought us lifesaving procedures, especially in emergency care. We just ask the question: What is our most effective option that causes the least amount of side effects? For some, a medication may fit these criteria and be a tool within their wellness toolbox. But a lot of the time, pharmaceuticals are not the best choice, but the only choice offered.

Are we going to defend doing the same thing repeatedly, expecting a different result? Just as is true with rejecting diet culture and anti-diet culture sentiment, we in functional medicine realize it doesn't always have to be "either-or" healthcare— either conventional medicine or alternative medicine. Often the best solution for your health is "both-and," the best of both worlds.

The same patriarchal system that criticizes functional medicine also shames and delegitimizes people struggling with chronic health problems like autoimmune conditions. So many people, especially women, are not listened to whenever it comes to their health. They aren't taken seriously, and they are often not listened to in mainstream medicine. The implicit systemic delegitimization of people when it comes to their health (and so much more) is one of the saddest things to witness. This is what I call *medsplaining*—kind of like mansplaining, but produced by a medical doctor with a god complex.

With medical gaslighting, patients are told, "Don't confuse your Google search for my medical degree." In response to that, I would say doctors shouldn't confuse their medical degree with your intuitively knowing your body and wanting to be both informed and heard when you advocate for yourself. My heart and passion has been consulting with people around the world who are doing everything their doctor tells them to do and everything they are "supposed" to do but are still struggling with health issues, don't know why they feel the way that they do, and are shamed for asking any questions about their health. They are told by their doctor in so many words that "It's all in your head" or "You are just depressed." Tell me, who wouldn't feel a little depressed when you know there is something going on with your body and no one is listening to you? People with autoimmunity, chronic fatigue, brain health problems, or hormone imbalances aren't crazy or hypochondriacal. Listen to your body, even if your doctor won't listen to you. Trust your intuition. The good news is that in many ways that archaic age is ending. A new era is emerging, spearheaded by a sea of people who are informed, intuitive, and desirous of agency over their body. Their awareness and health are rising. But don't be mistaken: Wanting to live healthy and asking questions is a radical act in a society that feeds and profits from its own health problems.

The good news is also that with functional medicine, there is some hope. Functional medicine teaches us how to look at the body as one complex organism instead of as separate unrelated parts that each need their own specialist. And more important, it teaches us that the gut-feeling connection is not only real but also an integral part of overall health and happiness. Serving as a sort of "clinical organizer" for my patients, I integrate different protocols to untangle gut-feeling dysfunctions and I work with other experts in different fields to put the needs of the patient before our own egos.

As we move into the next chapters—where we start learning how to restore a healthy gut-feeling connection—and then into the Gut-Feeling Plan itself, know that the overall philosophy and many of the recommendations and tips and tricks come from functional medicine, which I hope will be the standard of care in the future.

CHAPTER 4

Is Shameflammation Sabotaging Your Health?

So far we've talked about the physiology of the gut-feeling connection and how Shameflammation can be born from emotional suffering and a lack of mental healthcare. But let's be honest, many of us aren't walking around thinking that our levels of Shameflammation feel high on a certain day. No, most of us are more concerned with the very real physical symptoms that are affecting our health today, right now. How can you be sure that your health problems are caused by Shameflammation?

If your emotional world is sabotaging your physical one, it can present in symptoms that range widely from the obvious symptoms of diagnosed chronic health conditions to harder-to-pin-down symptoms like fatigue, sugar cravings, brain fog, and insomnia. My friend and fellow functional medicine leader Dr. Mark Hyman often uses the term *FLC syndrome,* or "feel like crap syndrome." When something is out of whack with our emotional world—ranging from our stress levels to past trauma to a lack of self-compassion—it can sabotage parts of our body in ways that seem awfully far from our gut or our brain.

The reason for this lies with our nervous system and hormones, which create the web of communication within our body. Our hormones are extremely susceptible to changes in our gut or brain, a fact that can help us understand why our health suffers when we don't take care of our body and mind. This neuro-hormonal system draws a straight line between our emotional world and our physical one. A dysregulated gut-feeling connection leads to the dysregulation of our nervous system, our hormones, and just about every other system in our body.

In this chapter, we'll be delving into some of the most common health problems I see in my practice, including how these are connected to the gut and brain and what we can do to repair this intricate internal ecosystem when it starts to go haywire.

The Gut-Brain-Endocrine Axis

Hormones are chemical messengers that send signals to and from different parts of the body. They're sort of like the body's internal communication system—and as we know, communication is everything. Oftentimes we think of hormones as pertaining only to reproduction—we hear the word *hormone* and we immediately think of sex hormones like testosterone, estrogen, or progesterone—but the truth is, hormones rule many aspects of your health, including your sleep-wake cycle, energy levels, sex drive, metabolism and weight, skin, blood sugar, and response to stress.

When you have issues with your gut-brain connection, your hormones are often the first thing to get knocked out of whack. As the master agents of communication in the body, your hormones are highly sensitive to the smallest internal changes. They are always conscious of what's going on around them, always attempting to maintain balance, and always adapting when something is off. They have an amazing ability to sense when things aren't quite right in the body and are quick to go haywire. Most important, they aren't able to just keep doing what they're supposed to be doing if something in the body isn't functioning the way it should be, even if it's happening far away from them.

This tendency for hormones to react to small shifts in the body occurs on something called the *gut-brain-endocrine axis*. This axis is incredibly sensitive to your emotions, stress levels, and changes in your nervous system like chronic sympathetic activation. For example, when the body is in that sympathetic activation vagal state—also known as fight or flight—it directly impacts the gut-brain-endocrine axis, lowering neural output of the brain and hindering its ability to communicate with the entire hormone system.

If your hormones aren't in balance, you'll constantly feel like you're swimming upstream when you try to make healthy lifestyle changes. Without healthy hormones, you'll be racked with fatigue, craving sugar, struggling with sleep, and unable to maintain a healthy weight. When I see patients with any of these symptoms, I always conduct comprehensive hormone testing to see what might be going on.

For the purposes of this book, we'll dive into a few of the major hormone systems of the body, how they are connected to the gut and brain, and how the Gut-Feeling Plan is going to help you get back on track.

Blood Sugar Imbalances and Metabolic Issues

Chances are that you or someone you know has a blood sugar problem. The statistics are shocking. Sadly, seven out of the top ten causes of death for Americans are chronic diseases, and most of them are tied to dysfunctional blood sugar.[1] Over 120 million Americans have prediabetes or diabetes, and nine of the ten leading causes of death in the United States are caused or worsened by metabolic dysfunction. There are an estimated 96 million Americans with prediabetes; 70 percent of these people will be diabetic within ten years, and 84 percent of people with prediabetes do not know they have it.[2]

All of these blood sugar issues come back to one hormone called *insulin*, which is responsible for taking the sugars from the foods you eat and shuttling them into your cells, where the sugars can be converted into energy to power your body. When you eat a food high in sugars or carbohydrates, especially when it doesn't contain much fiber, that food is quickly converted into sugar in your bloodstream, triggering the release of insulin to take the sugar out of your blood and send it to your muscles and cells to be used right away or to your liver to be stored for when you need it later. But here's the thing: You need only so much glucose, and if you eat a lot of sugar-rich and carb-rich foods all the time, your body may have trouble keeping up with the demand.

Unfortunately, eating too many sugar- and carb-rich foods is the norm in our society. The consequence is insulin resistance, which is when your body builds up a tolerance to insulin. In response, your body needs to produce more and more insulin to try to get the glucose in your blood into your cells. If your body can't keep up and it develops insulin resistance, you get chronically high blood sugar or type 2 diabetes.

The blood sugar problem in our country isn't a secret. You're probably already aware of the dangers of diabetes and what you need to do to prevent it. What isn't common knowledge is the fact that blood sugar health is intricately connected to our gut, our stress levels, and all the systems we've talked about so far in this book. Currently, there's a great focus on high blood sugar being caused by too much sugar intake, but the truth is that the causes of diabetes are more complex than that and are intricately related to the gut and our stress levels. You can draw many lines between blood sugar health and the gut-feeling connection. In fact, your gut health plays a key role in blood sugar regulation and insulin resistance. A study from the Center for Individualized Medicine at the Mayo Clinic followed a group of three hundred people over the course of six days. The researchers tracked glycemic responses to foods and found that they could only accurately predict blood sugar between 32 and 40 percent of the time when they took into consideration simply what foods the subjects ate and how many calories they consumed. But when the scientists factored in the specific composition of the microbiomes of participants, they were able to accurately predict blood sugar response 62 percent of the time.[3] Other studies also support the connection between blood sugar and the microbiome. Those who are overweight or have trouble losing weight—a symptom of underlying metabolic problems—tend to have lower microbiome diversity, with fewer beneficial microbes and more harmful bacteria and fungi.[4] In another fascinating study, scientists were able to transplant the microbiome of diabetic mice into healthy mice to make them diabetic as well—without changing what the mice were eating at all.[5] It's also been postulated that changes in the gut microbiome lead to metabolic issues, which lead to a type of low-grade chronic inflammation that puts you at risk for obesity and diabetes.

Now, I can't move on from the topic of insulin without talking about negative emotions, since there's a clear connection between the two. These days, stressful events like family losses or trouble at work are well known to be risk factors for triggering the onset of diabetes. In addition, studies have shown that traumatic experiences, family chaos, and behavioral problems during childhood are also linked to diabetes. So what explains this connection? It turns out that the main stress hormone, cortisol, causes blood sugar levels to go up. Technically, this is an evolutionary adaptation. When we're trying to fight or flee, we need immediate sugar in our blood to fuel our muscles and cells to get out of a dangerous situation. It therefore makes sense that when we encounter a threat, our body does what it's designed to do, stopping digestion and other less critical bodily processes, like repair and cleanup mechanisms, and funneling its resources to the heart, brain, and muscles. The only problem occurs when stress is chronic. Too much cortisol for too long can lead to chronically high blood sugar, which can contribute to diabetes and insulin resistance.

If you've got a blood sugar issue, I'm sure that your gut-feeling connection is playing an important role in your imbalance, and that healing will require an approach that tackles both the physical causes of blood sugar imbalances—such as gut microbiome imbalances and excess sugar intake—and the emotional ones, such as chronic stress or the effects of trauma. Luckily, the 21-Day Gut-Feeling Plan is designed to do precisely that.

Thyroid Problems

Unlike other hormones such as estrogen or even insulin, our thyroid hormones aren't something many of us think about much during our lifetime—that is, until there's an issue with your thyroid and you find yourself thinking about it all the time! The thyroid is a butterfly-shaped gland located on the front of the neck, and the hormones associated with the thyroid gland—there's a whole group of them that work together to regulate your thyroid function through a complex web of feedback loops—play a key role in metabolism, mood, temperature regulation, and other aspects of your health. When there's a problem with thyroid function, it can cause a wide range of symptoms. For example, low thyroid function, or hypothyroidism, which affects one in eight women in their lifetime, can cause weight gain, fatigue, and depression.[6] The most common cause of low thyroid function is the autoimmune condition called *Hashimoto's thyroiditis,* which occurs when your immune system starts attacking your thyroid, but you can have non-autoimmune thyroid issues, too.

As a functional medicine practitioner, I see thyroid health issues all the time. In fact, they're one of the most common issues I see in my practice, especially after a period of acute stress. Like insulin and estrogen or progesterone, thyroid hormones are extremely sensitive to stress and your psychological state. Research also shows that poor neurotransmitter expression and mental health issues like depression, anxiety, and bipolar disorder can be linked to hypothyroidism, and people with depression are known to have higher rates of thyroid conversion impairments.[7] As it turns out, as is true in the case of blood sugar health, your main stress hormone, cortisol, can sabotage thyroid health. Many of my patients discover that their thyroid problems started after a stressful time in their lives. As the authors of one study explain, the evidence suggests that stress hormones act on a certain type of immune cell—called a *T cell*—which shifts the activity of the immune system dangerously toward autoimmunity.[8] What I find in my practice is that many, many patients develop a thyroid issue after a physically or psychologically difficult time, such as going through a difficult pregnancy or childbirth, grieving, or starting their own business.

Thyroid hormones are also directly linked to gut health. For example, low thyroid function can reduce the movement of your intestines and leave you with sluggish digestion and poor elimination.[9] Not to mention, a significant percentage of thyroid hormone conversion happens in the gut, and an imbalanced, unhealthy microbiome can inhibit this process. Poor thyroid function also compromises your body's ability to absorb nutrients. Healthy thyroid function dampens gut inflammation, so low thyroid function can be linked with gastric ulcers and leaky gut syndrome. Thyroid health and blood sugar health are also intricately connected: For example, when your thyroid hormones are low, it decreases your ability to absorb glucose, which can cause chronic fatigue and insulin resistance.

Even more confusing is the fact that conventional doctors don't test all your thyroid hormones to look for an issue, which means thyroid problems are often missed. This leads to thousands of patients with underlying thyroid issues going untreated and undiagnosed for years and even decades at a time, while their doctor tells them that their lab results are "normal." In functional medicine, we look at the full picture of thyroid health and have higher standards for what an optimally functioning thyroid looks like. If you've got a thyroid issue, a gut-feeling approach is key; in fact, I'd say that the fastest way to heal your thyroid is to address your stress levels and gut-feeling connection.

Anxiety and Insomnia

Melatonin and cortisol are two of the most important hormones in our body. Every single day of your life is regulated by fluctuations in these two hormones. Here's what I mean: Every morning, your cortisol levels spike, and this gives you the energy to get out of bed and get your day started. Later in the day, when the sun starts setting, cortisol levels start to fall and melatonin production ramps up. This makes you feel relaxed, heavy-eyed, and ready to head off to sleep. This daily cycle of cortisol and melatonin is also known as your sleep-wake cycle.

Knowing that insulin and thyroid hormones are connected to the gut, you won't be surprised to find that melatonin and cortisol are intricately related to the gut-feeling connection, too. Some fascinating research out of Israel showed that the gut microbiome of mice changes throughout the day, thanks to these hormones. The study showed that when the mice were asleep, the gut microbiome shifted in ways that encouraged DNA repair and cell growth, and when they were awake, the gut shifted to promote detoxification and environmental sensing. The same seems to be true for humans—you're dealing with a surprisingly different gut environment depending on the time of day or night. Thus it makes a lot of sense that your digestion can get wonky after a long trip or a late night. Another study showed when the gut's circadian rhythm was disrupted by inducing jet lag in the mice, it left them more susceptible to gut infections like salmonella. There's also plenty of evidence that your gut microbiome regulates your sleep-wake cycle through the gut-brain axis.[10]

Many of us take the amazing coordination between these two hormones for granted—that is, until you pull an all-nighter or travel through multiple time zones and get jet-lagged, which can lead to fatigue, insomnia, mood changes, cravings, and brain fog. The daily rhythm between melatonin and cortisol can also get disrupted for reasons less obvious than an all-nighter or a long flight, such as by using electronics late at night, which signals to the brain that it is still daytime, triggering the production of cortisol at night and hurting melatonin production. This sleep-wake cycle can also be upset by chronic stress. When the body is chronically pumping out stress hormones, it can mess with your ability to get appropriate spikes and dips of melatonin and cortisol, which leaves you feeling somehow both chronically amped and anxious but also chronically fatigued and foggy-brained. Why is this? Because cortisol and melatonin play a role in more than just the sleep-wake cycle. Cortisol has the important job of regulating blood pressure, blood sugar, cardiac health, inflammation, and energy levels. Melatonin is more than just a sleep hormone. It's also an incredibly powerful antioxidant and anti-inflammatory hormone that is key to preventing disease and keeping us healthy as humans.

Now, I think we can all agree that none of the symptoms above sound like something we'd like to experience, but I want to take a minute to talk about the first one on the list—the ability to fall and stay asleep. Not getting enough sleep—in fact, simply not getting enough high-quality sleep—can be a major contributor to physical health issues. Sleep is when we recharge and reset our body and our mind. It's what allows us to have the resilience to tackle all the challenges of the day. If we want to maintain a healthy vagal tone and keep ourselves out of a chronic sympathetic state, we have to sleep, and we have to sleep well. Sleep might seem like a passive activity, and many people think they can skimp on it to be more productive during the day, but the truth is, the period that you are asleep is a very active time in your body and brain. During sleep, our brain is working to store the new information that we took in during the day. Our brain cells talk to each other, get organized, and regroup for the next day. It's also the time when the body and brain get rid of toxic waste and repair cells, a process called *autophagy* that is crucial for cancer prevention and longevity. During sleep, our muscles repair themselves, new proteins get synthesized, hormones are released, and new tissues grow.

Most important, sleep has an enormous impact on emotional health. Especially during rapid eye movement (REM) sleep, our brain processes emotional information, thoughts, and memories. Research shows that lack of sleep is extremely damaging to the way we store memories but especially to the retention of positive ones, because while we're sleeping, our brain favors the consolidation of positive memories and allows more neutral memories to fade.[11] What a powerful realization! Lack of sleep can make it harder to remember the good things and be a positive, optimistic person. Talk about a trigger for Shameflammation! Sleep also plays a big role in processing trauma; for example, one fascinating study showed that if we sleep within the first twenty-four hours after a traumatic experience, it can help us process and integrate the memories effectively and prevent the development of PTSD. And unfortunately, sleep problems are incredibly common, affecting between 50 percent and 80 percent of adults in the United States, especially those with mental health conditions like anxiety, depression, or ADHD.

The sleep-wake cycle is so important I could write an entire book on it, but for now, just know that in order to have a healthy body and mind, healthy cortisol and melatonin production is nonnegotiable. This isn't just because of the hormones themselves, but because, when you're not sleeping well, it immediately sabotages your mental fortitude and ability to make healthy decisions during the day.

Hunger and Cravings

Have you ever gotten bad news and lost your appetite? Have you ever found yourself snacking through a stressful day, always looking for the next sweet or salty or carby thing to put in your mouth? Have you ever felt sad, lonely, or misunderstood and had the urge to distract yourself from those feelings with comfort foods? If you said yes to any or all those questions—congratulations! You're 100 percent human. Our hunger levels, cravings, and taste buds are intricately connected to our nervous system, brain, and gut-feeling connection. This isn't anything to be ashamed or feel embarrassed about—our bodies were designed this way. Our need for food is so wrapped up in our other basic human needs, like those for love, community, pleasure, and understanding, that it only makes sense that we would have these tendencies.

So far in this chapter we've been diving into the ways that major aspects of your physiology are related to the gut-feeling connection, and your hunger hormones are no different. Two hormones in particular, called *leptin* and *ghrelin,* are the hormones largely in charge of your hunger and satiety signals and the overall energy balance in your body—which is a fancy way of saying how much energy you consume and burn each day. For example, leptin (also known as the satiety hormone) is made by fat cells that send signals to the brain to decrease your appetite. Leptin is largely responsible for your hunger levels over the long term. Ghrelin is a hormone that does just the opposite, signaling to your brain that you are hungry and need to eat. When these hormones are working in harmony, you get hungry when your body needs more fuel, and you get full when you've had your fill.

Unsurprisingly, both leptin and ghrelin are influenced by your gut. Studies have shown that certain bacteria decrease the sensitivity of leptin and predispose you to metabolic issues and weight gain.[12] Studies also show that stress can increase ghrelin production and decrease leptin production, predisposing a person to overeat.[13]

This delicate interplay between leptin and ghrelin is something I talk to my patients about all the time. Many patients come into my office frustrated by the knowledge that they can't seem to lose weight or stop eating the foods they know aren't the healthiest for them. They feel like they're always swimming upstream. Many of them have also been diagnosed with an inflammatory disease or an autoimmune disease, which makes them feel even more disconnected from their body and out of control.

With these patients, my approach always involves a multistep process that includes decreasing chronic inflammation through shifts in diet and lifestyle and a focus on the emotional factors that contribute to emotional eating and cravings. Oftentimes these patients are able to get their hunger signals back on track in no time with this holistic approach to hormone health, and I'll be sharing some of these practices in the 21-Day Gut-Feeling Plan in chapter 7.

Detoxification

You know when you're doing a little midweek cleanup or spring cleaning, and you walk around your house or apartment selecting things to throw away, donate, repurpose, or recycle? This is the way you periodically clean up your environment and make sure things stay fresh, healthy, and happy in your home. Well, your detoxification system is a lot like that; essentially, it helps you get rid of the substances that no longer serve your body.

The idea of a detox is something that often gets criticized as something akin to crash dieting. And I'll be the first to admit that there's no shortage of gimmicky fasts and cleanses that can do more harm than good. But the true ethos of detoxification is nothing like that; in fact, true detoxification is more about what you do eat than what you don't eat.

When I talk to my patients about detoxification, I explain it this way. Our metabolic processes create a type of waste that the body must process and get rid of, similar to the clutter that builds up in your living space over time. This includes waste from natural bodily processes—like when we produce hormones or repair our cells—and waste created from the foreign toxins and chemicals that we encounter in the outside world. You can think of your body's detoxification system like a sort of all-purpose compost-recycling-garbage crew that picks up that waste, packs it up, and then figures out what to do with it. Unfortunately, our world is full of toxins that threaten our health.

Most detoxification happens in the liver, which is why you've likely seen all types of liver detoxes advertised on the internet. In fact, almost everything you consume—anything from alcohol to over-the-counter medications to many of the ingredients in the food you eat—has to be filtered by the liver at some point. Detoxification occurs in two main phases. The first phase involves identifying the toxins lingering in your system and converting them to a form that makes them easier to remove, and the second phase involves neutralizing those identified toxins so they can be excreted from the body. Both phases of detoxification must be functioning properly to feel your best; for example, if phase 1 functions well but phase 2 is sluggish, the intermediate metabolites will build up, which can make you feel less than ideal. Unfortunately, supporting detoxification isn't as simple as avoiding toxins, because whether we like it or not, we encounter toxins every single day. These toxins disrupt the very foundation of our health—they upset the microbiome, they cause chronic inflammation, they majorly disrupt our hormones, and they overwhelm our detoxification system. The most common toxins include pesticides, herbicides, heavy metals like mercury, lead, and aluminum, phthalates found in beauty and personal care products, flame retardants found in furniture, electronics, and baby products, and biotoxins such as those from mold (mycotoxins).

Now, I'd never tell you that it's possible to avoid *all* toxins, but trying to decrease your exposure to toxins in your life is one of the best things you can do to help repair the gut-feeling connection. But here's the tricky part—the toxins we encounter aren't all chemical, pesticide, or pollution-based. In fact, by far the most insidious toxins we encounter daily often come from our own head in the form of chronic stress, negative emotions, and shame. They can also come from the people around us in the form of unhealthy, toxic relationships. These types of toxicities can affect your body and contribute to physical health problems just as readily as a toxin from your cleaning or cosmetic products. When you're in chronic sympathetic activation, your body goes into a fight-or-flight state and starts channeling its energy to the brain and muscles to prepare you to fight or flee; as a result, it neglects other important bodily processes, such as digestion, immunity, hormone balance, and detoxification. When you're in chronic fight or flight, it's like there's glue in the gears of your liver's detoxification mechanisms, and every step of detoxification is affected negatively. What do I mean by that? When you're stuck in a negative cycle, your body not only becomes more inefficient at detoxification but actually creates *more* toxins. Research shows that during times of stress or after a trauma, the body produces more damaging compounds called *free radicals,* which threaten to damage your cells and overwhelm the body. As a result, the toxins your body encounters every day start building up, and you start to feel the effects of that toxic buildup pretty darn quickly.

This is just one of the reasons why in my practice, detoxification isn't thought of as something we do just once or twice a year. Instead, I like to tell my patients to make their life a cleanse. This means eating detoxifying foods and nutrients, getting their sweat on, and drinking filtered water, but it also means constantly evaluating other types of toxicity that are less obvious, such as toxic productivity, relationships, or even positivity. If you're not sure exactly what that looks like in practice, don't worry. We'll be dipping our toes into this during the 21-Day Gut-Feeling Plan.

The world of hormones is wondrous, isn't it? I've been studying the human body for years, and hormones are still a source of constant fascination in my life. In some ways, they remind me of the bacteria in our gut—responding to everything you eat, do, feel, and think. If you are curious about your hormone, metabolism, gut health, and detoxification biomarkers, consider having lab work done—my telehealth center runs them for people around the world.

I know what we've learned in this chapter can be a lot to wrap your head around, but the most important thing to remember as we move forward is that this connection we've been learning about between the gut and the brain affects all aspects of your health. Everything in the body is connected. In fact, I like thinking of your body's internal system as an intricate fabric, delicately woven with different colors and patterns that together create a seamless, beautiful textile. Unfortunately, that also means that once part of your health goes awry, it's bound to knock others out of whack. It's sort of like when you get a snag in a new sweater: You know in your heart that that one thread popping out isn't where the problem is going to end, and pretty soon the issue spreads.

But here's the good news: Once we're aware of this, we can take our power back. Instead of allowing these health imbalances to spin out of control and sabotage our health and happiness, we can start to tame them and create a healthy ripple effect that breaks the vicious cycle for good.

How to Tame Shameflammation and Get Your Health Back on Track

At this point, you are basically an expert in the physiology of the gut-feeling connection and know how emotional and physical health are dependent on each other. You also understand the root causes of Shameflammation and are aware of how it can make its home in your body by exacerbating existing health issues and sabotaging your hormones. At the end of the day, we need all parts of our body to be working together in harmony to allow our bodies and minds to get fully back to a state of peace and calm.

My guess is that many of you have been dealing with some level of Shameflammation for years. The effects can be subtle—such as knowing that chronic stress plays a role in your health issue, whether it be headaches, IBS, or PMS—or extreme, when you feel like your heart and mind are all but disconnected from your body or you are diagnosed with an autoimmune condition, depression, anxiety, or chronic pain or fatigue. I see this often with patients with past trauma or those dealing with chronic health issues like autoimmune disease. These factors can act like a wedge in our gut-feeling connection.

So now that we know how Shameflammation occurs, what it looks and feels like, and how it affects our gut-feeling connection and our health, you're probably wondering: What's the secret to fighting it? The key to taming Shameflammation lies in feeding both our bodies *and* our minds the good stuff. We have to slow down, get still, and tend to the gut-feeling connection. This means a new approach to eating and thinking.

1. Feed your gut and your brain by eating a nutrient-rich diet.
2. Feed your head and your heart with self-compassion, stillness, and daily moments of mindfulness and relaxation.

This, not so coincidentally, is what the next two chapters are about.

CHAPTER 5

Feed Your Gut and Your Brain

Now, as a functional medicine practitioner and nutrition expert, you know I couldn't write a book without doing a deep dive into food and nutrition. There are situations where an elimination diet or other food or fasting protocols can be a helpful tool and one that I recommend. That said, the goal has never been nor will it ever be to whittle down the list of "good" foods to nothing but air, ice cubes, kale, and tree bark. The goal is to have a healthy gut that can tolerate all types of exciting, flavorful, diverse foods. In this book we are talking about nutrition in the context of feeding the body and the mind, which means focusing on a sustainable, enjoyable approach to optimal *health and happiness*. This nutrition advice in the Gut-Feeling Plan is designed to optimize the relationship between your physical and emotional health and infuse your lifestyle with a whole lot of simplicity and self-love. But before we get there, I'd be remiss if I didn't dive into the very real science behind nutrition and how it supports your gut-feeling connection.

So, although we've spent significant time so far talking about how wellness is about way more than food, we're not going to ignore food completely. Food can be both a cause and a solution to the problem of a dysfunctional gut-feeling connection. Repeatedly choosing to eat foods that don't love you back is like staying in a toxic relationship and wondering why you are still miserable. Choosing not to eat foods that don't love you back isn't restrictive—it's self-respect. The plain truth is that some foods can raise inflammation, mess up your blood sugar, hurt your digestion, and make you feel fatigued, anxious, or down. Diet culture is when your decision to eat something is laden in shame and obsession. Diet culture is about thinness, not health. Loving yourself enough to find out what your body really loves and needs for vibrant wellness is the ultimate body positivity. Accepting your body as it is doesn't mean you are settling for where you are right now. You are simply shifting your perspective toward making choices out of self-respect and self-love, not out of restriction, shame, obsession, or punishment.

Every new cell of your body is formed from the foods you consume. These nutrients (or a lack of them) are intimately interwoven into every part that makes you, you—your skin, brain, hormones, immune system, hair, genes . . . all of it. So the foods we are focusing on in this plan are superstars at supporting gut health, mood, brain health, detoxification, hormone health, and healthy inflammation levels. They are the best foods to get your body into a parasympathetic state.

In this chapter, we won't be pushing an all-or-nothing approach to food. What we'll do is cover the foods that cause health issues and spend a lot of time celebrating the foods that heal your body.

So, setting aside obsession or a pressure to eat the "perfect" diet, let's talk about how different foods influence our health and our happiness.

The Foundation of a Stress-Free Food Plan

Food is indeed a powerful influence over your biochemistry and over your gut and feelings, but you aren't likely to get much information about this kind of "prescription" from your conventionally trained doctor. Today in U.S. medical schools, students on average receive only about nineteen hours of nutrition education over their four years of school, and only 29 percent of U.S. medical schools even offer med students the recommended twenty-five hours of nutrition education.[1] A study reported in the *International Journal of Adolescent Medicine and Health* assessed the basic nutritional and health knowledge of medical school graduates entering a pediatric residency program and found that, on average, they were able to answer only 52 percent of the eighteen questions correctly.[2] In short, most doctors would fail a basic nutrition exam because they simply don't have the necessary training in this field.

It's highly ironic that nutrition is such a low priority for mainstream medicine, since a staggering 80 percent of the chronic diseases mentioned above are completely preventable and reversible with lifestyle choices. Functional medicine is a large part of filling these gaps created by conventional medicine and our health culture.

A stress-free food plan is all about having the most impact with the least amount of restriction. Most foods are on the table, and I'll only recommend taking a close look at how certain foods make you feel so you can make informed and conscious choices. The world is so focused on labeling foods and diets (and ourselves) that we've left no room for nuance, context, personalization, intuition, or flexibility. We haven't left any room to be patient and kind with one another, forgiving one another, and forgiving ourselves. We really haven't left any time to pause and ask ourselves, *Is the way I'm eating and living making me happy? Am I even enjoying the food I'm choosing to eat?* As you can guess, all this conflict and noise contributes to only more stress and confusion.

At its core, nutrition and lifestyle medicine should be about bringing people peace—starting with what, when, and which foods they eat. But all this confusion has left people stressed out and feeling like they're constantly missing something or doing something wrong. Allow me to offer a little clarity.

Protein—The Stable and Reliable Friend

If there's something that most nutrition and health experts can agree on, it's that protein is at the core of any healthy diet. When you're eating to tame Shameflammation, you can think of protein as your steady and reliable friend—the one who always has good advice, is great at planning ahead, and keeps you thinking clearly when you might otherwise spin out. Protein is the foundation of any good diet, especially one that is meant to support your health and happiness.

Protein and the amino acids that make it up are what help us feel satiated and what build muscle, cartilage, skin, and bone. It's what repairs our cells and tissues when we get injured or age, and it keeps our metabolism functioning, helping us burn fat and maintain a healthy weight. The list of protein's benefits is practically endless. We all need it, and when we don't get enough, it doesn't take long before our body starts to feel the effects. For example, too little protein can affect brain functioning and mental health because neurotransmitters are made from amino acids. For example, dopamine (known as the "pleasure" chemical) is made from the amino acid tyrosine, and serotonin (known as the "happy" hormone) is made from tryptophan. If you lack either of these two amino acids, there could be a suboptimal production of serotonin and dopamine, which can lead to a low mood and even aggression.

So what's the healthiest source of protein? You probably already know that there's a lot of back-and-forth about the best sources of protein, especially among the paleo/keto/carnivore and vegan/vegetarian crowds. The best sources of protein are the ones that *you* love to eat, align with your values, make you feel satiated, but also love you back.

Animal-Based Protein

Animal protein is often criticized, but when done correctly, animal products can be excellent sources of protein. Here are some high-quality sources of animal protein:

- Eggs (6 grams of protein per egg)
- Wild-caught salmon (17 grams of protein in a 3-ounce serving)
- Beef (22 grams of protein in a 3-ounce serving)
- Bison (24 grams of protein in a 3-ounce serving)
- Chicken (21 grams of protein in a 3-ounce serving)
- Lamb and mutton (23 grams of protein in a 3-ounce serving)
- Organ meats such as liver (23 grams of protein in a 3-ounce serving)
- Venison (26 grams of protein in a 3-ounce serving)

When evaluating any food, consider not only its nutrient value but also how much you enjoy it and whether it aligns with your values. Maybe quinoa and beans aren't the most bioavailable sources of protein, but if they're what you love and they make you feel good physically, then they should be on your list. There are a ton of healthy protein sources to choose from. We often think that getting enough protein requires us to eat chicken breast at every meal, but as you'll see below, nature provides us with a bunch of plant-based sources of protein.

Plant-Based Sources of Protein

NUTS AND SEEDS
- Almonds (6 grams of protein per 23 nuts)
- Brazil nuts (4 grams of protein per 6 nuts)
- Cashews (4 grams of protein per 18 nuts)
- Chia seed (4 grams of protein per 2 tablespoons)
- Flaxseed (4 grams of protein per 2 tablespoons)
- Hazelnuts (4 grams of protein per 21 nuts)
- Hempseed (11 grams of protein per 3 tablespoons)
- Macadamia nuts (2 grams of protein per 11 nuts)
- Pecans (3 grams of protein per 19 nut halves)
- Pine nuts (4 grams of protein per 165 nuts)
- Pistachios (4 grams of protein per 49 nuts)
- Sacha inchi seeds (9 grams of protein per 40 seeds)
- Walnuts (4 grams of protein per 14 nut halves)

Don't forget about nut and seed butters. They're a great way to infuse your day with some protein. For example, almond butter has 6 grams of protein per $1/4$ cup of butter, which means slathering some on a banana or dropping some in a smoothie can give you a nice dose of plant-based protein that doesn't require much prep or cleanup.

PROTEIN IN VEGETABLES
- Artichokes (4 grams of protein per $1/2$ cup)
- Asparagus (2.9 grams of protein per cup)
- Avocado (2 grams of protein per $1/2$ avocado)
- Broccoli (2 grams of protein per $1/2$ cup, cooked)

- Brussels sprouts (2 grams of protein per $^1/_2$ cup)
- Peas (9 grams of protein per 1 cup, cooked)
- Spinach (3 grams of protein per $^1/_2$ cup, cooked)
- Spirulina (4 grams of protein per 1 tablespoon)

OTHER PLANT-BASED PROTEIN SOURCES
- Hemp protein powder (12 grams of protein per 4 tablespoons)
- Hempeh (tempeh made from hempseed) (22 grams of protein per 4 ounces)
- Maca powder (3 grams of protein per 1 tablespoon)
- Natto (organic non-GMO) (31 grams of protein per 1 cup)
- Nutritional yeast (5 grams of protein per 1 tablespoon)
- Sacha inchi seed protein powder (24 grams of protein per 4 tablespoons)
- Tempeh (organic non-GMO) (31 grams of protein per 1 cup)

When we dive into the 21-Day Gut-Feeling Plan, we'll be reflecting on our protein intake and whether we're getting too much or too little. But for now, just remember that protein equals stability. It's there to keep you grounded, and when you're working on reestablishing a healthy gut-feeling connection, staying grounded is everything.

Fats—The Secret Source of Energy

Speaking of stability, the other secret to lasting energy and a stable body and mind is healthy fat, which in recent years has finally gotten the attention and appreciation it deserves as a macronutrient. Finally, the days when we counted grams of fat and looked for the words *fat-free* on labels are gone. In fact, healthy fats are now one of the most praised macronutrients.

Fat is essential for our hormone health, healthy inflammation levels, and a flexible metabolism. It's also essential to brain health, and not getting enough fat can impact cognition, mood, and behavior. Fat is an essential part of every cell in our body. One long-term study that analyzed data from over 12,000 people over ten years showed that men on a low-fat diet were 26 percent more likely to be depressed after one year than men consuming enough fat. The same study showed that women on a low-fat diet were 37 percent more likely to be depressed after one year than other women. These numbers remained high ten years later.[3]

That said, it's not as simple as stocking up on fatty foods—because not all fats are created equal. And when you hear the words *healthy fats*, it can be hard to know exactly what that means. The healthiest types of fats are called *monounsaturated fats* (or MUFAs). MUFAs include olive oil and avocado oil, which are both liquid at room temperature but become solids when left in the fridge. MUFAs have been shown to support heart health and healthy cholesterol levels as well as reduce the risk for stroke, diabetes, and visceral belly fat, which we know is the most damaging type of body fat. MUFAs are also key to great mental health.

The next type of fat is called *polyunsaturated fats* (or PUFAs). PUFAs can be a little bit confusing because the health benefits of a PUFA depend on how it's made. There are natural PUFAs, like those found in fatty fish and nuts and seeds, and then there are more processed PUFAs like canola, soybean, and vegetable oils. A Harvard Health article explains that supplementing with a type of PUFA called *omega-3 fatty acids* is being studied as a treatment for various mood disorders and psychiatric conditions, such as postpartum depression, schizophrenia, borderline personality disorder, obsessive-compulsive disorder, and attention deficit hyperactivity disorder.[4] Foods like fatty fish have been associated with optimal brain health, while industrial seed oils have been associated with just the opposite—more specifically, with worsened memory and decreased learning ability.[5] We'll talk more about oils later in this chapter, but for now just know that PUFAs are somewhat complicated.

Then, there are *saturated fats*, which open a whole new can of worms. In my last book, *Intuitive Fasting*, I wrote that if PUFAs are the most confusing type of fat, saturated fats are the most misunderstood. Well, I stand by that statement. You've probably heard that saturated fats should be avoided because of their link to heart disease, but the truth is that saturated fats—like those in butter, coconut oil, eggs, and meat—are not quite as dangerous as we've been led to believe. Recent studies have shown that the association between saturated fat, cholesterol, and heart disease isn't as clear cut as we thought.[6] What we know now is that cutting out saturated fats and lowering cholesterol aren't the be-all and end-all for a healthy heart. We also know that saturated fats are key to healthy inflammation levels, healthy hormones, healthy cells, and a healthy brain. We won't go too far into this research here, so just know that consuming saturated fats shouldn't keep you up at night. The amount of saturated fat you should ideally consume each day depends on your genetics, energy needs, and the composition of the rest of your diet (for example, if you combine sugars and saturated fats in the same meal, saturated fats can make the sugar even more unhealthy than it already is).

There is one type of fat that you should try to avoid entirely called *trans fats*. Trans fats often appear on food labels as hydrogenated or partially hydrogenated oils and are often hiding in processed and packaged foods like peanut butter, margarine, creamers, spreads, and even cookies, cakes, and potato chips. They're also frequently used by fast-food restaurants, which is just another item on a long list of reasons to avoid fast food as much as you can. Eating trans fats is like taking the express path to inflammation and health issues, and such fats are also associated with an increased risk for diabetes, obesity, and heart disease.[7]

If you're feeling overwhelmed by all the different types of fat, just remember that the most important thing is to know which fats are healthy; that way, you can eat those, and this will naturally crowd out the other stuff. So, without further ado, here are the best fats for getting your gut-feeling connection back on track.

FOUNDATIONAL FATS: FATTY FISH + SEAFOOD
+ Alaskan salmon, wild-caught
+ Albacore tuna (U.S./Canada, wild, pole-caught)
+ Anchovies
+ Atlantic mackerel
+ Catfish
+ Cod (Alaskan)
+ Flounder
+ Herring
+ Lobster
+ Mussels
+ Oyster

- Rainbow trout
- Rockfish
- Sardines
- Shrimp
- Sole (Pacific)
- Yellowfin tuna (U.S. Atlantic, wild, pole-caught)

FOUNDATIONAL PLANT-BASED AND VEGETARIAN FATS
- Pasture-raised eggs
- Olives and olive oil
- Raw or sprouted nuts and seeds
- Avocado and avocado oil
- Full-fat dairy products, especially raw or fermented
- Grass-fed butter and ghee
- Coconut oil
- Goat cheese

Carbohydrates—*Not* Your Mortal Enemy

If you've read anything about nutrition lately, there's a good chance you left thinking that carbs are your mortal enemy. As has happened many times before—such as when we vilified anything with fat in the 1980s and 1990s—we're currently in a phase of making *carbs our mortal enemy.* But I want it on record right here and right now that carbs are not your enemy. While I agree that as humans, we are eating way too many carbs on average—mostly in the form of added sugars, refined grains, and simple carbs—carbohydrates aren't inherently bad. In fact, when it comes to your health and happiness, carbs are pretty darn important. Let me explain.

Carbs make you happy. And I'm not talking about the consumption of mass amounts of sugar or white bread making you feel good at the moment. Carbohydrates help your body produce important brain chemicals like serotonin. Answer me this: Have you ever tried to cut out carbs and felt anxious and sad or been so amped at night you can't sleep? That could be due to the sudden decrease in carbohydrates.

Serotonin plays a key role in your nervous system and in your ability to sleep; it fends off negative thinking and anxiety. There is even a strong connection between carbs and sleep, because serotonin is made from carbohydrates but melatonin— also known as your sleep hormone—*is made from serotonin.* Therefore, some people try to cut out all carbs too quickly or for too long and end up staring at the ceiling at night, overcome by anxious thoughts. Pretty interesting, isn't it?

Fruits and Vegetables—Fiber and Polyphenols

Fruits and vegetables are full of beneficial nutrients, antioxidants, and beneficial fibers that feed your gut and your brain, which means a healthier gut-feeling connection. Study after study shows that if you want a healthy gut and a healthy brain, these plant-based foods are key. For example, a systematic review that analyzed the results of almost 6,000 studies found that people with a high total intake of vegetables and fruits seem to experience higher levels of optimism and self-efficacy.[8] This may be the first time you're hearing the word *self-efficacy,* but it means "an individual's belief in his or her capacity to execute behaviors necessary to produce specific performance attainments," as defined by the American Psychological Association. In other words, eating your fruits and veggies is linked to a higher likelihood of believing in your own strengths and abilities. That gives new meaning to the phrase *plant powered,* doesn't it? Even more, the same review showed that high fruit and vegetable intake is associated with lower levels of psychological distress and depressive symptoms. Another study showed that people who eat at least 470 grams of fruits and vegetables a day had 10 percent lower stress levels than those who consumed only half of that amount. For reference, 470 grams of blueberries is about 2.7 cups![9]

The sneaky but great thing about fruits and vegetables is that the more of them you eat, the less room you have for the other stuff, like refined sugar and inflammatory oils. As you'll see in chapter 8, the foundation of all the recipes in this book is made of colorful fruits and vegetables. Why? Because they really *are* the key to a long and healthy life. And the good news is that, unlike with carbs and fats, it's hard to go wrong with fruits and vegetables. In fact, the key to healthy fruit and veggie intake is consuming a diverse array. Why? Because the bacteria in your gut feed off the fibers, called *prebiotic fiber,* found in these plant-based foods. A study published in *Nutrients* showed that a diet rich in vegetables and other high-fiber plant-based foods improves gut bacterial diversity within two weeks.[10] I find that patients who are trying to heal their sensitive guts often do better at the beginning with more soft, cooked vegetables, like soups and stews. Digesting food requires a lot of energy, so this makes it easier for your gut to process everything and focus on healing instead. Even fruits can be cooked down into a compote, making them gentler on a healing digestive system.

We tend to focus on the potential pitfalls of carbohydrates, like how they can spike your blood sugar or be addictive, while ignoring the clear benefits of having some type of carb in your diet. The key to healthy carbohydrate intake is to focus on healthy, nutrient-rich carbs over empty, blood-spiking carbs like simple sugars and refined grains, which is what we're doing in the 21-Day Gut-Feeling Plan. For patients who have blood sugar problems, macro-stacking can be a great way to bring clean whole-food carbohydrates into your meals. Macro-stacking involves consuming carbs, such as fruit or potatoes, *after* fiber-rich vegetables, proteins, and fats. In this way, you can buffer any blood sugar spike that can happen even with healthy carbs.

Below you'll find a great list of healthy fruits, vegetables, and gluten-free grains. These foods are high in antioxidants, fiber, and some whole-food-based carbohydrates that are key to a stress-free diet.

VEGETABLES

- Alfalfa sprouts
- Artichokes
- Arugula
- Asparagus
- Bean sprouts
- Beets
- Bok choy
- Broccoli
- Broccoli sprouts
- Brussels sprouts
- Cabbage
- Carrots
- Cauliflower
- Celery
- Chard
- Chives
- Collard greens
- Cucumber
- Dulse
- Endive
- Ginger
- Jicama
- Kale
- Kelp
- Kohlrabi
- Kombu
- Leeks
- Lettuce
- Mushrooms
- Nori
- Okra
- Olives
- Peppers

- Radishes
- Rhubarb
- Rutabaga

- Scallions
- Seaweed
- Spinach

- Swiss chard
- Turnips
- Water chestnuts

FRUITS
- Apple
- Avocado
- Blackberries
- Blueberries
- Cantaloupe
- Cherries
- Clementines
- Eggplant
- Grapefruit
- Grapes

- Guava
- Honeydew melon
- Kiwi
- Lemons
- Limes
- Lychees
- Mangoes
- Oranges
- Papayas
- Passion fruit

- Pear
- Persimmon
- Pineapple
- Quince
- Raspberries
- Star fruit
- Strawberries
- Tangelos
- Tomatoes
- Watermelon

STARCHY VEGETABLES
- Acorn squash
- Butternut squash
- Carrots

- Peas
- Potatoes
- Sweet potatoes

- Yams

LEGUMES
- Black beans
- Edamame
- Fava beans
- Garbanzo beans
  (chickpeas)

- Great northern beans
- Green beans
- Kidney beans
- Lentils
- Mung beans

- Navy beans
- Peas
- Pinto beans
- White beans

GRAINS
- Gluten-free oats
- Quinoa
- Rice

Herbs and Spices: Nature's Pharmacy

As we wind down with the foundations of a stress-free diet, I'd be remiss if I didn't take a second to talk about herbs and spices. These foods are like the cherry on top of a great diet and lifestyle. They provide a ton of flavor, a ton of health benefits, and they are cheap and easy to use. In the recipes in this book, you'll see how I love to experiment with herbs and spices to infuse plant healing into not just teas and elixirs but also meals and snacks.

HERBS

- Basil
- Bay leaf
- Chiles
- Cilantro
- Cumin
- Dill
- Lavender
- Lemon balm
- Mint
- Oregano
- Paprika
- Parsley
- Rosemary
- Sage

SPICES

- Allspice
- Anise seed
- Annatto
- Caraway
- Cardamom
- Celery seed
- Cinnamon
- Clove
- Coriander
- Cumin
- Fennel
- Fenugreek
- Garlic
- Ginger
- Horseradish
- Juniper leaves
- Juniper berry
- Mace
- Mustard
- Nutmeg
- Paprika
- Peppercorns
- Poppy seeds
- Sea salt
- Sesame seed
- Star anise
- Sumac
- Turmeric
- Vanilla bean (no additives)

We made it! I hope the last few pages felt like a real celebration of food. At the end of the day, food should bring us joy. Just think about the abundance of healthy foods on this planet, waiting for us to enjoy.

CHAPTER 6

Feed Your Head and Your Heart

The tools in this chapter are all uniquely included to be a part of your parasympathetic toolbox. We'll be using these tools in the Gut-Feeling Plan to rebuild the connections between body and mind. They are all different ways to nourish your gut-feeling connection, regulate your nervous system, and tame Shameflammation.

As we learned earlier, chronic stress, trauma, and shame can cause us to feel separate from our bodies and constantly disillusioned with the messages it sends us. This is no way to achieve a sense of ease in your life; in fact, it can lead to a vicious cycle that takes us further and further from inner peace, driving a deeper wedge into the gut-feeling connection. Not feeling connected to our bodies can cause massive stress, exacerbate mental and physical health issues, and leave us constantly worrying, questioning, and on edge.

But here's the good news. There are some science-backed secret antidotes to all this emotional and physical stress and suffering.

Slow Down and Embrace the Joy of Missing Out

The first tool in feeding your head and heart is something I like to call JOMO, or the joy of missing out. This metaphysical meal is a way of life. Many of us are quick to feel left out. With social media making it incredibly easy to post only the most carefully curated version of our lives, it's no surprise that seeing everyone's filtered highlight reel makes us feel like we're constantly missing out on something bigger, better, and more fun. I have seen firsthand how much stress and anxiety FOMO (the fear of missing out) can cause, and how that heightened stress response can trigger health problems and exacerbate symptoms. That's why I believe it's more important than ever to embrace the antithesis of FOMO—JOMO.

During times of stress, your body's stress hormone, cortisol, is on high alert. Even though this is a normal response, chronically high cortisol levels are not and may lead to a whole slew of health problems. Instead of saying yes to every little thing, commit only to the things that are the most important to you, those that are in line with your overall values and goals. Your time is sacred. Allow yourself space to breathe without always feeling on edge.

I know that you can't always control your packed schedule, but I do encourage you to try inserting some time for stillness. Chances are, the busier you are, the more likely you are to grab whatever is easiest and quickest to eat. Between work, social events, volunteering, and family activities, you have little time to prepare meals. But the more you edit down your schedule, the more time you have to pay attention to the food that you are putting into your body. A JOMO lifestyle can give you more opportunity to grocery shop, cook, and sit down to a real meal instead of eating on the go. Whether you are eating a relaxing meal by yourself or sharing it with loved ones, you'll have time to slowly chew your food, enjoy the flavors, and give your gut a chance to fully digest whatever you are eating. Embracing JOMO will free up your time for personal growth because you are no longer bound to a schedule of what you think you *should* be doing. Instead, you'll be able to do what you *actually want to be doing*. And the more you find fulfillment in your own journey, the less you'll feel left out of what others are doing.

We all have people in our lives who consistently disrupt our peace. You know, the people who always have something negative to say about your life and seem only to bring you down with their words and actions. Your interactions with people can take many forms—from close relationships you've had for years to encounters with trolls on social media. When you finally start embracing JOMO, those who aren't true friends of yours will weed themselves out of your life very quickly. Basically, if you aren't around to serve them, they will quickly lash out or forget about you and move on. And the less time you give to social media (because remember, you are enjoying your personal growth journey), the less time you'll spend being berated by online trolls. We've talked a lot about how emotions and stress can build up over days and months and years. Well, JOMO gives us a chance to regularly reflect on what is going on in the present moment. With a more mindful outlook on life, you can take the time necessary to unpack anything from your past—good or bad—and use it to make the best decisions for your present and your future.

Turning FOMO into JOMO is one of the best ways to calm stress and anxiety. With all the noise online and inside our minds, you need to create spaces of stillness both within and without. You'll be amazed what you have time to do when you can tap into the joy of missing out, such as investing in some of the different "metaphysical meals" in this chapter to feed your head and heart and support your parasympathetic nervous system.

Allow Self-Compassion to Flourish

For most of human history, our stress came from threats like being chased by predators and hunting for food to survive. Of course, even in our modern, relatively comfortable society, we can often use a little more of the grit of our ancestors, despite the fact that in most cases, our stressors these days are tamer and rarely relate to our immediate survival.

But one layer of our modern problems is unquestionably worse today. Over the long term, our chronic stressors are turning out to be the demise of our health. The rat race of today, with its deadlines, time stressors, 24-hour news cycle, perpetual hyper-connection through social media, and poor sleep is severely damaging our well-being.

Over time, humans have adapted a physiological pattern called the *conserved transcriptional response to adversity* (CTRA). This is a type of gene expression that's associated with increased inflammation. So if you were being chased by a predator, CTRA allowed for some helpful short-term benefits, such as increased healing, physical recovery, and the increased likelihood of your survival. But in ancient times, humans weren't constantly being chased by large predators or human enemies. The stressful times would eventually calm down and allow the body to recuperate.

Now, with our modern mental and emotional stressors rarely turned off, our body constantly thinks it's being chased by predators. As a result, long-term activation of our brain's CTRA is contributing to chronic inflammation and increasing the risk of health problems.[1]

Because of CTRA and other stressors, our emotional stress is a chase that never ends, and it's wearing on our brains and bodies. A study published in the journal *Clinical Psychological Science* found that self-compassion had a very real impact on our health. People in the study who were asked to focus on their bodily sensations, as well as those told to think kind thoughts toward others and themselves, had lower heart rates and a lower sweat response at the end of the experiment. Unsurprisingly, the participants who were encouraged to think critically about themselves had a faster heart rate and greater sweat response.[2] The findings suggest that being kind to oneself switches off the threat response and puts the body in a state of safety and relaxation important for regeneration and healing.

Instead of complaining either in your head or out loud, try speaking love into your life. About 37 trillion cells are intently listening to how you speak to them. Speak kindly. Words and thoughts are powerful modulators of your biochemistry.

Acceptance and self-compassion can fight chronic inflammation from stress and in turn help decrease the risk of health problems. This is the immense power that your thoughts and emotions have over your health. I see so many people who eat perfectly but remain unwell in part due to the unhealthy emotional pain and stress they are holding on to. Forgive yourself and forgive others.

The highest, most noble battle you will ever wage is the war between what you feel and what you know deeply, beneath the feelings. The more you like yourself, the less you need others to like you. Learning to love yourself is a journey, but it's a beautiful one, with ups and downs alike. One of the side effects of our new breed of chronic stress is the mental and emotional alienation from our true selves and others. We get lost in our own minds, consumed with a constant stream of obsessive and repetitive thoughts, and fail to develop habits—such as mindfulness meditation and yoga or to taking breaks from social media—that bring peace and calm into our lives. Sometimes the best form of healing is acknowledging the role you play in your own suffering and showing yourself grace and compassion to evolve from that awareness. In short, you are not your negative thoughts and emotions. Take them captive and observe them for the transient things they are. Build a healthy relationship with yourself. True sustainable wellness flows from realizing your intrinsic worth.

And finally, when you cultivate more compassion for yourself, you can show compassion to others more abundantly. It's easy to reflexively judge something or someone we don't understand, especially when we are exponentially harder on ourselves. True compassion says, "I don't understand this or it's not for me, but I see the humanity in this person and show kindness anyway." Otherwise, we become what we hate in others: judgmental, hateful, shaming, small-minded, and militant. Kindness, compassion, and empathy are nothing more than empty words and vapid virtue signaling until you can show them to people you disagree with or don't understand.

Should Everyone Be in Therapy?

Many of us are resistant to starting therapy, and this is understandable. As much as things have changed over the years, there's still a stigma about what going to therapy means. Many of us think that going to therapy means that we have a mental health condition, aren't strong enough to handle things on our own, or have some sort of inherent emotional weakness. But that isn't true, not even a little bit. In fact, those who attend therapy are typically more emotionally resilient, aware, and able to maintain healthier relationships.

The other modalities mentioned throughout this chapter are all incredible ways to nurture your head and your heart. That said, if the sections on trauma or multigenerational trauma resonated with you, there are other practices to know about that can help you process your emotions and heal past wounds. Counseling with a professional therapist is one route that I always suggest to my patients, and thanks to telemedicine, seeing a therapist is easier than ever. Many people have questions about the benefits of therapy, and it can be scary to bring to the surface emotions that you've long tried to avoid feeling or to recall memories that you've long tried to forget. As someone who collaborates with mental health specialists in patients' care, I can tell you that therapy has helped countless of my patients reclaim their lives. We've learned that our body stores the stress and emotion we feel and that when this builds up, it often expresses itself in the form of physical health issues, like autoimmune disease, chronic inflammation, a thyroid issue, or hormone imbalances. Therapy can help reverse this cycle and allow your emotions to move through you.

There's one type of therapy that's particularly fascinating for past trauma, including those suffering from post-traumatic stress disorder (PTSD). It's called *eye movement desensitization and reprocessing* (EMDR), and it was developed in the 1980s by a psychologist named Francine Shapiro. As you can guess from the name, this type of therapy is centered around eye movement— specifically, that certain eye movements make it easier to process distressing events or emotions. With EMDR, you work with a professional to dive into negative thoughts or experiences and pair them with specific eye movements that can help the brain reframe these experiences. Since the first study in the 1980s showed that EMDR can be successful, interest in this therapy has exploded over the years. According to the EMDR Institute, as many as 90 percent of those with trauma have a significant reduction in PTSD symptoms after just three sessions. EMDR was originally developed for treating trauma and PTSD, but it can also be successful for panic attacks, anxiety disorders, phobias, eating disorders, addiction, and depression.

So what explains the wild success of this strange therapy? The mechanisms behind EMDR are still a bit of a mystery, with experts hypothesizing anything from the eye movements' ability to synchronize the two brain hemispheres to how the movements are similar to rapid eye movement (REM) sleep, which is when the brain consolidates and properly stores memories. Whatever the explanation, of the more than 500 brands of psychotherapy existing in this world, EMDR stands out above the rest and is recommended by organizations like the World Health Organization, the American Psychological Association, and the Department of Veterans Affairs. EMDR has helped many of my clients overcome trauma, limiting beliefs, and negative thought patterns as well as psychological health issues like anxiety and depression.

When you start slowing down and getting mindful, it's only natural that some negative thoughts, either toward yourself or others, will come up. This makes total sense, as slowing down tends to allow thoughts and feelings that are just beneath the surface float to the top. When this happens, it's a great opportunity to practice forgiveness. As is true of all the practices in this chapter, forgiveness can have a positive impact on both your psyche and your physical health. For example, one study tested the effects of forgiveness on the brain using functional magnetic resonance imaging (MRI). The participants were asked to imagine social scenarios or emotionally hurtful events; then they were asked to either forgive the supposed offenders or harbor a grudge against them. The results showed that forgiveness was associated with a much more positive emotional state and strengthened parts of the brain that involve cognition and empathy.[3] This simple act will lower inflammation and cortisol levels and shift the body into more of a parasympathetic state: rest, repair, digest, balance.

We know it benefits us physically and mentally to forgive others, so imagine how powerful it is to forgive yourself. Treating yourself with forgiveness is one of the foundations of fending off Shameflammation and achieving optimal health and wellness; that said, I know it's not as simple as it sounds. Your relationship with yourself is the longest, most consistent relationship of your life, and there are bound to be ups and downs, regrets, self-criticisms, and things you wish you could change about yourself, from your body to your behavior and habits. The key to forgiveness of yourself lies in compassion—more specifically, in a philosophy called *mindful self-compassion*. Ancient philosophical traditions have long put forth this type of compassion as a sort of antidote to suffering. More recent research suggests the same. The benefits of mindful self-compassion are impressive; studies have shown that those who practice this type of compassion are happier, with greater motivation, relationships, and physical and mental health. They are also more psychologically resilient when coping with traumatic events.

So how do you practice self-compassion? The next time you're facing a challenge—a day filled with anxiety, criticism at work, or a difficult situation involving another person—talk to yourself the way you know a supportive friend would. Tell yourself what you need to hear instead of piling on by blaming or further criticizing yourself. Instead, comfort yourself and provide yourself with the emotional support that you need. Don't do this quickly. Instead, allow yourself to bask in the feeling of directing compassion and empathy toward yourself, allowing the feelings to sink in.

Slow Down and Reconnect with Your Gut Feelings

I know you've heard of mindfulness before, whether it be in the context of meditation, yoga, or something else. Mindfulness is a great method for getting us back in our bodies and in the present moment, which is especially important for healing the connection between your body and your brain. And luckily, there are about a million ways to become more mindful. So let's talk about some of my favorites.

Meditation

This method is like a magical antidote to Shameflammation and the physical symptoms it causes—and it's free, we can do it anywhere at any time, and it takes only a few minutes a day. Meditation includes a group of practices that together help calm all the inner noise, allowing your body and mind to spend some much-needed quality time together.

You've probably heard of mindfulness in the context of stress relief or anxiety, but in this book we're taking a slightly different approach, one that is tailored specifically to restoring the gut-feeling connection and influencing the way we store thoughts and emotions in our bodies. As Dr. van der Kolk wrote in his book *The Body Keeps the Score*, "Mindfulness not only makes it possible to survey our internal landscape with compassion and curiosity but can also actively steer us in the right direction for self-care."[4] Indeed, mindfulness seems to be the secret key to reopening the door between the mental and the physical. In recent years, research has revealed the true power of mindfulness for everyday people. Here are just a few examples of the power of mindfulness:

- A review of forty-seven trials involving 3,515 participants suggests that mindfulness meditation programs show moderate evidence of improving anxiety and depression; other studies have shown that it can be helpful for conditions like high blood pressure, chronic pain, and insomnia.[5,6]
- Mindfulness-based treatments may be effective in restoring connectivity between large-scale brain networks in those with PTSD, leading to a reduction in emotional over- and under-modulation common after traumatic experiences.[7]
- Studies have shown that mindfulness practices can lessen the symptoms of irritable bowel syndrome; in fact, one in particular showed that a year after implementing a mindfulness practice, patients showed significant reductions in abdominal pain, flatulence, and bloating.[8]
- Research shows that even brief mindfulness practices induce gray matter plasticity in the brain, which is associated with self-awareness and emotion.[9]
- Mindfulness practices can increase vagal tone, which is associated with positive emotions and feelings of goodwill toward yourself, by stimulating that famous vagus nerve we learned about earlier.[10]

As you can see, mindfulness is something that every single person can do and benefit from in one way or another. When it comes to fighting Shameflammation, investing in mindfulness is key.

So how do you do it? The cool thing about mindfulness is that there are countless ways—many of which we'll be experimenting with in the Gut-Feeling Plan—to slow down, quiet the noise, and allow our gut-feeling connection to restore itself. Modern life encourages us to get lost in our own minds, not to mention in the great river of information to which we are exposed almost every minute. Many of us are constantly consumed with obsessive repetitive thoughts and negative self-talk.

There are a bunch of different types of meditation, but most involve sitting quietly in a comfortable position (for example, cross-legged or in a chair with a straight back) and bringing your attention to something specific, whether that be your breathing, your body, the present moment, or an intention. Meditation is probably the most direct way to get into the present moment, and that's likely why the research on meditation is so robust.

Most of our stress comes from the way we respond to an event. Meditation has a way of dissolving the negativity and resistance around a given situation.

Because of this, meditation is one of our most powerful tools for restoring that gut-feeling connection; and luckily, there are a bunch of different types of meditation to try out:

◆ **Mindfulness Meditation.** This type of meditation encourages the meditator to focus on the sensations that come up in the present moment, including thoughts and emotions, and just observe what occurs without judgment.
◆ **Body Scan.** Another popular type of meditation is a body scan, which involves bringing your attention to the top of the head and then bringing your awareness slowly down the body all the way to the toes.
◆ **Loving-Kindness Meditation.** In this type of meditation, you ground yourself in the present moment by focusing on cultivating the feelings of love, compassion, and kindness and sending them out into the world or to specific people or places during your meditation.

Meditation allows you to realize that you are the vast beautiful sky, not the passing clouds. Meditation is the deep knowing that you are not your thoughts, emotions, or current situation, which come and go like the weather. Interrupt anxiety and negative thoughts with deep breaths, stillness, and gratitude.

Being at peace with all outcomes is a place of immense power. The concept of *nonattachment*—that is to say, dissolving attachment to and identification with impermanent external things or people—is one of the biggest concepts that meditation has taught me. Love, peace, joy, and liberation originate from within. I have a long way to go to master this, but strengthening your awareness so as not to overvalue outcomes, things, and how people make you feel provides deep wellness. Instead, honor and have gratitude for things or people as they come and go, without making them part of your identity and sense of worth.

The great news is that the more you meditate and heal, the more you will grow tired of the unhealthy things in your life. Your relationships, food choices, and habits will start to change the more you heal. Junk becomes intolerable. As you practice meditation and the other tools in this chapter and throughout this book, you will begin to attract and surround yourself with high-vibration people: the kind, the grateful, the uplifting, the open-minded. These people inspire others to level up their life while still letting others know that they are loved and accepted exactly where they are now. You yourself will be growing into that kind of person.

The people who say, "Mindfulness just isn't for me" are usually the ones who need it the most. It is sort of like saying, "Exercise is not for me." Work that mindfulness muscle. Find a practice that you can stick with and be consistent with.

Breathwork

Breathwork might seem like a strange concept if you're a beginner to mindfulness. I mean, aren't we all breathing all the time either way? The truth is that the *way we breathe* can greatly affect our inner and outer environment, and specific breathing techniques can be like a fast track to calming the nervous system and getting in the present moment. Have you ever noticed that when you're stressed or anxious, you start taking shorter, faster breaths? Have you ever noticed that these breaths tend to be sharp, and that you breathe mostly into the chest and shoulders, which start to tense up? Well, mindful breathing encourages us to take deep, slow breaths into our bellies instead of our chests. So when I use the word *breathwork*, I'm talking about taking advantage of this connection by intentionally changing the way you breathe to bring about a change in your physical and mental state.

Some of my favorite breathwork exercises include:

- **For Beginners—Diaphragmatic Breathing.** As I mentioned before, many people end up breathing into their chest and shoulders instead of their diaphragm. This means that the best place to start getting into breathwork is to focus on breathing from the diaphragm in order to restrengthen the muscles there until such breathing becomes second nature. To practice diaphragmatic breathing, lie flat on the floor with one hand on your chest and the other on your stomach. Breathe in through your nose for 2 seconds, making sure your stomach expands rather than your chest. Next, purse your lips and exhale for 2 seconds while pressing on your stomach. Repeat a few times and notice any sensations you feel. It may take some time for you to get used to this type of breathing, so don't be discouraged if you don't experience any obvious benefits the first few times! You may even feel a bit light-headed.
- **Intermediate—4-7-8 Breathing.** You may have heard of the 4-7-8 breath before. This technique is a way to build on the diaphragmatic breathing above. The best part about this breath is that you can do it anywhere, even while you're on a call for work, out for a walk, or stuck in traffic. To try it out, breathe in for a count of 4 seconds through your nose. Hold your breath for 7 seconds, and then exhale slowly for 8 seconds through your mouth.
- **Intermediate—Box Breath.** Also known as *square breathing*, this more forceful breathwork practice became popular with Marines and athletes for its ability to help you feel relaxed while still giving you a boost of energy. Inhale through the nose for 4 seconds, hold your breath for 4 seconds, exhale from your mouth for 4 seconds, and end by holding your breath for 4 seconds. Repeat this four times.

- **Advanced—Holotropic Breathwork.** Another type of breathwork that is helpful in taming Shameflammation is called *holotropic breathwork. Holotropic* means "moving toward wholeness," and such breathwork is designed specifically for emotional healing, self-exploration, and empowerment. Thus it's no surprise that this method is perfect for reestablishing the gut-feeling connection. This type of breathwork is more advanced than any of the ones above and involves breathing at an increased rate for as much as an hour. This changes the balance of oxygen to carbon dioxide in the body and is thought to produce an altered state of consciousness, similar to psychedelics. Holotropic breathing is generally done in a group setting, lying down with your eyes closed, with a professional who guides you through the process. It can also be done in pairs, with each person alternating between assuming the role of the breather and the sitter. As you breathe, you dive into your own psyche and release unwanted emotions, thoughts, and patterns. This type of experience can be transformative, but I recommend building up to it by experimenting with some of the other breathwork methods first.

Breathing exercises have been part of traditional healing systems for centuries. For example, in the yogic tradition, breathing is called *prana,* which means both "breath" and "energy." The Old Testament Hebrew word *ruach,* means "spirit" and "breath," with the Holy Spirit (Ruach HaKodesh) literally translating as "the holy breath." In traditional Chinese medicine, breath is intricately linked to *qi,* which is known as the life force of the body that flows through channels in the body, corresponding to specific organs, health conditions, and even emotions. There's substantial research that breathwork does actually change our physiology. For example, a study on the 4-7-8 breathing technique showed that it not only helped improve breathing in COPD patients but also led to a decrease in anxiety and depression.[11] In fact, this technique has demonstrated an ability to reduce asthma symptoms, reduce fatigue, bolster stress management, reduce hypertension, lessen anxiety, reduce aggressive behavior, and improve migraine headaches.[12] Other studies have shown that diaphragmatic breathing led to improvements in sustained attention, mood, and cortisol levels.[13] Seems like it's worth a try, doesn't it?

Yoga

As a person living in the twenty-first century, you have more than likely tried at least one yoga class in your life. The philosophy behind yoga—which can be traced back to northern India over 5,000 years ago—is all about uniting the mind and body and spirit. In fact, the Hindi word *yoga* means "to yoke," which means "to join or harness." Thus it will come as no surprise that yoga can be a helpful tool for restoring the gut-feeling connection. In fact, researchers have drawn some fascinating connections between polyvagal theory and yoga philosophy. For example, the neurophysiological states of polyvagal theory line up mysteriously with the concept of gunas in yogic philosophy. Gunas are known as the main energetic forces of the universe that determine our physical and emotional state:

1. Tamas, which represent the energetic forces of chaos and darkness
2. Rajas, which represent activity and passion
3. Sattvas, which represent harmony and presence

As the authors of one study explain, "These two different yet analogous frameworks—one based in neurophysiology and the other in an ancient wisdom tradition—highlight yoga therapy's promotion of physical, mental and social well-being for self-regulation and resilience."[14]

The parallels between yogic concepts and polyvagal theory may help explain why the list of yoga's benefits is a mile long. I won't even scratch the surface, but yoga can increase self-esteem, lower stress levels, decrease chronic pain and reduce opioid use, relieve anxiety, and reduce depression (even in those that have not responded to medication).[15,16,17,18] Yoga is known to influence executive functions in the brain, which are responsible for regulating goal-directed behavior, our habits, and our emotional responses to situations. For me, yoga teaches that there is space between action and reaction; it teaches you to observe yourself in motion, notice your thoughts and tendencies when things get hard, and give yourself a little space to breathe and connect with your body.

Tai Chi

Like yoga, the ancient Chinese traditional practices of tai chi and qigong are like getting on the express train to a more united body and mind. Often described as "meditation in motion," these practices involve a series of flowing movements paired with deep breathing. These ancient practices have been proven beneficial in modern times, too. According to the Mayo Clinic, studies have shown that tai chi and qigong can lead to:

+ Improved mood
+ Increased energy
+ Increased quality of restful sleep
+ Improved immune system
+ Lowered blood pressure
+ Overall improved well-being[19]

So, what's the secret to all these benefits? Like yoga, tai chi and qigong seem to be able to target the autonomic nervous system. For example, one study showed that the practice led to an acute decrease in sympathetic activation—more than other types of exercise; another showed that tai chi was able to increase the strength of vagal modulation to tilt the nervous system toward a calmer, more connected state.[20]

Somatic Therapies

Meditation, breathwork, yoga, tai chi, and qigong as well as massage, grounding practices, dance, and drumming are all examples of modalities that are used in something called *somatic therapy*. Somatic therapies are based on the concept that the body stores trauma in all the cells of the body. All unexpressed emotions can have physical effects. This can leave the body stuck in sympathetic fight-or-flight inflammation mode, perpetually reliving the past. This can show up in many forms of gut-feeling dysfunction like chronic pain, autoimmunity, digestive problems, chronic fatigue, anxiety, depression, panic attacks, and PTSD. Somatic therapies focus on moving and releasing the tensions and stored, locked trauma in the body and sometimes talking through or cathartically meditating on what you are releasing. Studies have shown somatic therapies to be significantly beneficial at relieving symptoms of inflammation, chronic pain, and PTSD.[21]

Here is a simple at-home somatic therapy you can try on your own:

1. Unclench your jaw, relax, and lower your shoulders.
2. Release the tension in your body, shaking your arms out, opening and closing your fists, rolling your head around, and relaxing your neck.
3. Next, move your eyes up and down and left and right, relaxing them.
4. After this, open your mouth, stretching your jaw. Stick out your tongue to increase the stretch.
5. Now pat, tap, or squeeze all of your body all over with your hands. You can also do this by giving yourself a hug for as long as you need.

This and other somatic exercises will help to activate your parasympathetic nervous system, making you feel grounded, safe, calmed, and contained.

A Word on Psychedelics, CBD, and Microdosing

We've made our way through a long list of therapies and techniques for restoring a dysfunctional gut-feeling connection. Many of them have decades of research to support their ability to heal the head and the heart. There are also some emerging therapies that are worth knowing about. Psychedelics include drugs like LSD, ayahuasca, and psilocybin, the main active ingredient in psychedelic mushrooms, all cause changes in mood, perception, and the way the nervous system works, helping to shift the body more into a parasympathetic state.

You may have heard chatter about microdosing, especially if you've done any research on psychedelics. Microdosing is the practice of taking very small amounts of drugs with the goal of hopefully gaining the benefits of these drugs without getting high. Of course, at this point, microdosing psilocybin and other psychedelics is not legal in the United States except in specific research or therapeutic settings, and the FDA has not approved them for the general public as yet. That said, the research that has been done on psychedelics in a therapeutic setting has revealed some noteworthy and exciting benefits for people struggling with PTSD, resistant cases of anxiety and major depression, and some autoimmune conditions. To learn more about the therapeutic use of psychedelics in a clinical or research setting, I suggest looking at the work of the Multidisciplinary Association for Psychedelic Studies (MAPS).

Another area of research has to do with cannabis—more specifically a class of compounds called *phytocannabinoids*, which are found in the cannabis plant. CBD is my favorite cannabinoid for most people, since it's non-psychoactive, which means it won't give you a high or cause a bad case of the munchies, but it will still have beneficial effects on your health. CBD oil from organic hemp oil is also incredibly helpful for getting you out of the fight-or-flight state and back to a state of parasympathetic calm. I've seen the powerful impact CBD oil can have on anxiety, not only in my patients' lives but also in my own life. Multiple studies have found CBD oil to be an effective treatment for social anxiety and a natural anxiolytic (anxiety calmer).[22] CBD oil may have benefits similar to those of some of the common antianxiety medications, without the side effects. CBD oil can also reduce anxiety by increasing the activation of the prefrontal cortex and lowering activity in the amygdala—two areas of the brain involved in anxiety.[23] Animal studies also suggest that CBD can activate neurogenesis—the development of new neurons—in the hippocampus.[24] This works to activate CB1 receptors, which balance GABA and glutamate levels to reduce anxiety. I recommend starting with 20 milligrams of full-spectrum CBD and seeing how you feel. You can experiment with as much as 100 milligrams, a couple of times a day.

Healthy Boundaries and Healthy Social Connections

I've been doing this new cleanse. It's called the *unkind-people fast*. It's really helping my severe bullshit intolerance. I highly recommend it. Seriously, though, the people you spend most of your time with either build you up or feed into your negative thoughts, and you'll want to start cutting the latter group out of your social circle.

There should be three main groups of people in your life: (1) your inner circle of friends who mutually lift one another up; (2) people you can be a positive influence on; and (3) the outer circle—anyone who will negatively influence you. Keep your distance from these "energy vampires" who are constantly negative or make every conversation about themselves. Sometimes wellness looks like sending certain people out the exit door. In some cases, before fully cutting the relationship, try setting boundaries first. However, if that fails, it's time to say goodbye to toxicity. When an unhealthy relationship fizzles out, don't chase after it out of habit or insecurity. Honor that person for the lessons they brought you, but now is the time for cutting the toxic out of your life because that lesson is learned.

One of the first things to learn about setting boundaries is to not confuse empathy with unhealthy boundaries. I know you are good at it, but it's not your responsibility to carry others' pain or negativity. Empathy doesn't mean making someone else's problems your own. Quit watering people who don't want to grow. Stop trying to be everything to everyone. This is a hard pill to swallow for my fellow empathic friends out there, but we need to stop letting people who are at war with themselves influence our energy. We humans have energy exchanges all day, every day. The people we interact with—in person, on the phone, via text, email, social media, or even glances on the street—can all affect our mood, thought processes, and trajectory for the day. We need to create healthy boundaries, wherever possible, with people who try to pull others into their negativity and gossip.

It's easy to get caught up in complaining about someone for whom we find it hard to show compassion or understanding. Negative chatter and gossip have a way of eroding mindfulness and building a toxic relationship. Normalize not having to talk smack or gossip about someone to feel better about yourself. Quit using gossip as a way to connect with or bond with someone. Positive, functional relationships are good for your health. When you hear gossip, just walk away or try to change the subject.

One of the greatest things I've learned so far concerning boundaries, especially when it comes to social media, is to not take criticism from someone you wouldn't take advice from. Who you are and what you stand for develops over the course of your life, through your experiences and relationships. During that journey, you will likely come across people who have opinions on how you should behave, what you should wear, and what you should believe. Receiving unsolicited criticism from a person who has no real place in your life is the last thing you need to be doing. Sometimes wellness looks like asking yourself three simple questions:

- Does this person truly know me?
- Can I trust that this person has my best interests at heart?
- Has this individual been present for both my wins and my losses?

Running through this quick mental checklist puts words and opinions into perspective, revealing what should hold weight in your life and what should not. This simple process serves as a reminder that while constructive criticism from the right person can help you become a better version of yourself, sometimes it's best to just let words roll off you.

Every word we speak has the power to bring positivity or negativity into every environment and every conversation we're in. Think twice before participating in an argument: Will anything good and productive come from it? What solution are you looking for? Quit trying to convince someone who is committed to misunderstanding you. Beautiful things happen when you create a chasm between you and negativity.

Another essential lesson of setting healthy boundaries is to stop saying maybe when you mean no. Boundaries are medicine. Let *no* be your multivitamin. Use it as needed, sometimes daily. No response is still a response, and it's an immensely powerful one. Sometimes silence speaks volumes. The use of *no* is a healing balm and *because I don't want to* is a good enough reason. JOMO it up.

And finally, know that setting healthy boundaries isn't rude. Sharing your feelings isn't being dramatic. When this clicks, you will resonate on a whole different level, attracting all sorts of awesome things to your life. Realize that you don't have to dim your light to make others feel comfortable. You're not "too much." Stop believing that. Shine bright.

Having healthy boundaries and healthy social connections supports your parasympathetic pathway, leading to lowered stress hormones and inflammation, better gut health, and so much more.

The 4S Metaphysical Meal Plan

When I talk to my patients about repairing the gut-feeling connection, I often talk to them about infusing their day with micro-moments of stillness and nourishment. I call these *metaphysical meals,* because they're just as important as what you eat. You can eat the healthiest foods under the sun, but if you're serving your body a big slice of stress and shame every day, you are sabotaging all the good you are trying to do for your wellness. The philosophy behind the metaphysical meal centers on the fact that wellness isn't just about what you're eating at breakfast, lunch, and dinner, it's also about what you're serving your head and your heart.

Metaphysical Meal Meditation benefits your brain, your body, and your health and the connections between them all. It can be anything from practicing gratitude to taking a hot bath to having a good cry session. Metaphysical meals are key to the Gut-Feeling Plan because they show you ways to reconnect with yourself on a deeper level and nurture your head and heart. The Four Steps of the Metaphysical

Meal include stillness, sweetening judgment, setting intentions, and sealing your meal. Here's how it all breaks down into a 15-minute practice:

1. **Stillness.** As we just learned in the section on mindfulness and meditation (see pages 90–95) stillness is where it's at. For 5 minutes, take time to check in with your body and the thoughts or emotions you might be holding on to. This is where you can try out some of the techniques you learned in the previous sections by doing a body scan, a somatic exercise, or a breathing exercise as your way of entering the present moment.

2. **Sweetening Judgment.** Many of us spend a lot of time judging ourselves, judging others, or wishing we didn't feel the things that we do. Instead, let's practice having compassion for ourselves and others. As you sink into the present moment, feel compassion for yourself, your loved ones, and the world. As you strengthen this practice, cultivate the same feelings of compassion for those you have found difficult to love or forgive and see them as a child. As the saying goes, resentment is like drinking poison and waiting for the other person to die. Observe any thoughts and emotions that come up, even negative ones. Remember that these are just passersby; they aren't who or what you are. Allow yourself to spend some time just being still. Make friends with the present moment and make friends with yourself. Spend about 5 minutes diving into this loving-kindness meditation, cultivating self-compassion and compassion for others.

3. **Setting Intentions.** Now that you've reached a place of clarity and stillness, it's time to set an intention. This could be an intention for the day, for your life, or for others. If you want a more structured approach, you can write it down in a journal to make it feel more concrete. You can take about 2 to 4 minutes here.

4. **Sealing Your Meal.** You know when you enjoy a nice long dinner with friends or family? You take your time, and at the end of the meal you have a nice tea or coffee. This ritual acts like the cherry on top of a great experience. Well, I want you to do the same thing with your metaphysical meal. This can be a moment of gratitude to the universe, God, the source of life, or your higher

self. Anything that makes you feel like you're connected to something greater than yourself.

Metaphysical meals are all about making the mundane a meditation. That way you can infuse your day with many small moments of peace, gratitude, self-compassion, and other keys to mindfulness. In the Gut-Feeling Plan, we'll be doing a series of these metaphysical meals and experimenting with different ways to make the mundane a meditation.

CHAPTER 7

The 21-Day Gut-Feeling Plan

Your body is a beautiful temple, and this chapter is about bringing what you've learned so far together. I know you are all go-getters and you've probably been excitedly awaiting the moment when we get to put all the information you've learned into action. Well, I'm happy to report that in this chapter, you'll get to jump in and put some of these learnings to use. But let me warn you, this is not the typical go-go-go wellness plan that focuses on totally overhauling your routine and diet.

Why? Well, for one, whether you're a newcomer to wellness plans or a seasoned wellness enthusiast, those plans can be intimidating and take up a fair amount of your time and energy. Sometimes this is a necessary part of healing. For example, in the previous lifestyle plans I've written, such as the 4-Week Flexible Fasting Plan in *Intuitive Fasting*, I give specific instructions for what to eat (because no one should be trying to fast their way out of a poor diet). In *The Inflammation Spectrum*, I guide you through a tailored elimination diet, which hinges upon you eliminating all potentially inflammatory foods completely for at least four weeks, step by step. But these plans are specifically designed to help target underlying health imbalances that contribute to a wide array of diseases and dysfunctions. If you've already done the plans in my other books, consider this plan a peaceful, mindful reset where you have the chance to reflect, exhale, and tend to your body and mind. Here we use food as both a medicine and a meditation to calm our nervous system, regulating our gut-brain-endocrine axis.

But before we jump in, let's answer some questions I know you'll have about the plan. That way we can get the administrative work out of the way before we finally set off on our 21-day journey.

Common Questions Answered

Unlike other plans you may have done in the past, there won't be a strict list of things to eat and not eat, action steps to complete, or activities to avoid. Instead, we're going to spend these 21 days slowing down, getting quiet, and focusing on our gut-feeling connection.

What Can You Expect over the Next 21 Days?

Unlike my previous plans, the 21-Day Gut-Feeling Plan is broken down day by day instead of week by week. Each day will have an intention that we'll be focusing on that day, and then it'll be broken down into two subsections—the gut section and the feeling section. Both will include a teaching, challenge, action step, or moment for reflection. You'll recognize most of them, as we've covered them already throughout the course of this book. For example, you might be taking steps to optimize your daily melatonin-cortisol cycle, reflecting on your sugar intake and whether it might be contributing to Shameflammation, or experimenting with breathwork for stimulating the vagus nerve. Each day is a fresh, new opportunity to nourish and regulate your gut-feeling connection from the inside out and the outside in.

Will I Be Making Dietary Changes During the Gut-Feeling Plan?

Unlike the plans in my other books, the 21-day lifestyle plan is more of an explorative journey toward wellness than a prescription for it. I will teach you how to strengthen your intuition and discover your priorities and likes and dislikes. For example, on Day 3, instead of suggesting that you cut out all refined or added sugar for the duration of the plan, I encourage you to track your sugar intake and then reflect on which sources of sugar in your life are bringing you down. I've already made a pretty strong argument for consuming sugar, processed foods, and alcohol only in moderation to boost physical and mental health, but I'm not going to give you hard-and-fast rules about what to eat and what not to eat in this plan. It's up to you to decide what changes will help you the most. If you want to treat the 21 days as an opportunity to up your nutrition game, my suggestion is to look back at chapter 5 and stock up on the foods that make up a stress-free meal plan. That way, instead of focusing on eliminating any one food, you're primed to celebrate the foods that love your body back.

What About Recipes? Do I Have to Follow All of Them?

You know I couldn't write a book without including delicious, nutrient-rich recipes. All the recipes in chapter 8 will help you heal Shameflammation and contain ingredients that support the gut and the brain. You can stick to the food lists in chapter 5 and the recipes in chapter 8, but I want to be clear that *this is completely optional.* Feel free to experiment with whatever recipes speak to you throughout the plan. The recipes are divided into breakfast, lunch, dinner, desserts, and snacks to keep things interesting throughout the 21 days.

Who Will Benefit from the Gut-Feeling Plan?

The short answer is that I designed the 21-Day Gut-Feeling Plan for anyone and everyone. It works for those just beginning their wellness journey, but it's also great for those who feel burnt out or overwhelmed by their current wellness routine or by the overwhelming amount of wellness advice out there. You can think of this plan as a sort of detox from other more restrictive plans, a reset to begin healing your relationship with food and your body. It allows you to reflect and tune in to your inner knowing so that you can craft a sustainable lifestyle plan that works for you. Over the years I've learned that a few smart changes to a person's lifestyle can make a world of difference.

How Can I Prepare?

There's no required shopping or supplement list that you need to tackle before you begin. This plan is all about taking each day as it comes and being present throughout the 21 days. I do also give a few dietary and supplement recommendations that I think almost anyone can benefit from, but there's no need to buy those before the plan starts. For those of you that like to be extra prepared and organized, I'd recommend buying a notebook or journal to write down your thoughts and reflections throughout the plan. After you have completed the plan, I recommend keeping the notebook around to refer back to anytime you need to reconnect with that gut-feeling connection.

How Much Time Do I Need to Reserve Each Day?

The truth is, you can do this plan anytime, anywhere. In fact, there are days when it will take you only 5 to 10 minutes. This means that you don't have to wait for a month without weddings, trips, dinner parties, or holidays (as if that even exists) to start. This plan is designed to fit into your schedule. If you were waiting for the right time, it's now. I recommend reading the daily plan first thing in the morning, maybe over your favorite morning beverage. By carving out a few minutes, you can allow yourself time to reflect on the theme of the day and the gut and feeling items. Alternatively, you can read the day's content the evening before. Do what works for you!

What Are We Trying to Accomplish over the 21 Days?

My hope is that you infuse a beautiful grace and lightness back into wellness and discover what that means and how you get there, that you will have learned the art of being well. My hope is that by Day 21, you will see for yourself that your inner dialogue and emotional world are an integral part of your overall biology and physiology and vice versa. If you have a physically healthier gut and lower inflammation levels, you're going to feel better about yourself. I want to leave you feeling a little more confident about making your own decisions and a little freer to focus on your health and happiness instead of on all the rules about food and the conflicting advice being thrown at you from all directions. I want you to see the value in making healthy choices because you love yourself and want to celebrate yourself, not because someone gave you marching orders or you're trying to force your body into submission. Mostly I want to help you identify the low-hanging fruit in your life—in other words, the small things that make a *huge* difference in your overall health and happiness. In short, I want you to find Food Peace and Body Peace. A successful wellness practice is all about doing the small things that have a big impact and then not stressing about the rest.

Do I Have to Follow the Food Plan 100 Percent?

The Gut-Feeling Plan is about Food Peace, not falling back into beating yourself up or shaming yourself if you eat something that isn't serving you. If you choose to eat the cookie, eat it and enjoy it, and then move on. Don't hold on to it, don't be filled with guilt or shame, don't feel like you should just give up on eating healthily. Shame is worse than any cookie. Use the experience as a tool of self-reflection and mindfulness, a way to learn body talk. Did it serve you or not? Was it worth it? Use meals as a meditation just as much as you use them as a medicine to feel freaking amazing. The food plan includes the foods that are just the best, most delicious ways for you to serve your gut-feeling system. The plan is about discovering how to love your body enough to nourish it with delicious food medicine.

The concept of "cheating" when eating is antithetical to sustainable wellness. It is part of the spectrum of disordered eating that plagues our culture. Is the food you eat serving you or sabotaging how you want to feel? That is the question; it's not about moral judgment, failing, or virtue. If you choose to eat a food that doesn't make you feel great, do it rationally, neutrally. Observe how it makes you feel, learn from it, and move on. If it wasn't worth it, then you will grow in awareness for next time: You love feeling great more than you wanted something that made you feel like shit. This is an essential part of Food Peace.

The plan in this book is about learning to make this paradigm shift. It doesn't happen overnight. Give yourself grace.

Before we jump in, I just want to take a second to pause and admit to you that

I'm really excited about this plan. As I sit here writing, I'm imagining all of you reading these pages. I want you to know that I've written this plan with so much love and admiration for you. Taking steps to reflect on your health and happiness is courageous, and I want you to know that I see your bravery and I see you.

Okay, now let's get right into the 21 days together, shall we?

DAY 1

Food Peace Foundations

The time has come to heal, to move away from unhealthy patterns, and to break up with foods, people, and habits that don't love you back. I'm so happy you're here. In fact, I can hardly contain my excitement that you decided to join me on this journey. Thank you for trusting me with your time, energy, and health. For Day 1, we'll be starting with some simple but powerful intentions that act as a foundation for the rest of the plan.

A little context before we jump in: As a general rule, we focus too much on action items when it comes to our health. We talk about the newest exercise, the supplement we just started taking, the latest superfood we need to incorporate into our smoothie, or the 5-, 10-, or 30-minute meditation challenge we're planning to do just as soon as we have time. Now, I'm not saying that taking action is a bad thing—I wouldn't be writing a 21-day health plan if I thought that!—but I do believe this often ends with a lot of people on a hamster wheel, chasing a vision of "optimal" health that's always a little bit out of reach. I want to move away from a version of health that you'll accomplish only once you tick enough items off your to-do list or experiment with a thousand different options before hitting on the one miraculous routine. Today I want to tap into the fact that many of us already know what makes us feel good and what doesn't. And if we don't, sometimes all it takes is a little bit of quiet stillness for us to figure it out.

Gut: Identify One Food or Ingredient That Lowers Your Frequency

Instead of overhauling your entire lifestyle—which can make us feel discombobulated and even anxious—today take a few minutes to reflect and identify one food or food group that you already know doesn't mesh with your body but is still part of your regular routine. This could be dairy, which may leave you constipated, or it could be wheat bread, which leaves you fatigued and cranky. It could also be beans, which leave you bloated to no end, or it could be something like caffeine, which you know triggers your anxiety and sabotages your sleep. Refer to chapter 2 for a list of the most common foods and drinks that don't love people back very much. Now, here's the challenge that many of you (especially those self-proclaimed perfectionists or type A people) out there will face: You are *not* allowed to make a massive list of all the foods you think you shouldn't eat. Instead, pick one food that you *know* doesn't sit well with *your* body because you've seen concrete evidence of that in the form of physical symptoms. Next, and here's the other hard part, just reflect on that. You can ask yourself the following questions:

- How does this food make you feel?
- Why is it still part of your regular routine? Theoretically, could you replace this item with something else? Is there something you enjoy more that you could eat or drink instead?
- Could you simply consume less of that food or consume it less frequently? Avoid black-and-white thinking and resist telling yourself that you should never eat that food again.

This isn't an order or a prescription to eliminate this item entirely for the 21 days (although you can go ahead and do that if it feels right!). Instead, it's more of an awareness exercise to become more conscious of what makes you feel good and what doesn't.

Feeling: Do One Healthy Activity That You LOVE

For today's feeling task, let's focus on the positive. I want you to take a minute and think about a nonfood lifestyle practice that makes you feel great. This could be any activity of any duration—maybe it's 10 minutes of journaling, maybe it's 1 minute of belly breathing, maybe it's an hour of tennis or a quick walk around the block without your phone. For me, even just a few minutes of reading a physical book or a walk in nature makes me feel energized, inspired, and happy. Choose one thing that feels doable today and go do it! Afterward, I want you to really let the positive feeling you get after that activity sink in. This is a tip that I learned from Dr. Rick Hanson, a psychologist and researcher, as a way to help overcome the brain's negativity bias—that is, our tendency to quickly forget positive feelings and experiences and ruminate on negative ones, however small and infrequent they may be. This is just our brain's way of protecting us from harm, so we shouldn't beat ourselves up. Instead, we can try to override that bias by letting the feelings and experiences really sink in. Soaking up the great feelings we get from doing something uplifting for ourselves is like amplifying that experience, making it even better.

DAY 2

Take a Pause

I've already talked a lot about how much your feelings and emotions can influence your health. But here's the tricky part: Many of us struggle to give our emotions breathing room or find it hard to figure out what it is we're actually feeling at any given moment. Today is all about slowing down and giving your body and mind a little more breathing room.

Gut: Give Your Gut a Rest

Part of giving your feelings some room is working to minimize distractions and outside noise. And one of the biggest daily distractions is snacking. Don't get me wrong: I love a good snack, especially one that is high in protein and healthy fats and tides you over until your next meal. That said, snacking can keep our minds and bodies constantly distracted—not to mention keeping our digestive system constantly working to break down food—and create a lot of noise throughout our entire day. We often turn to food, especially the sweet or salty kind (or sweet *and* salty kind), to regulate our emotions and distract us from how we're really feeling. And as we know, sugar can actually influence your stress response and make you feel temporarily happier and calmer. So today I challenge you to take a look at your snacking habits and ask yourself if they are really serving you. Cutting back on snacking can improve gut health, safeguard blood sugar health, and leave a little more room for other things throughout the day. Now, I want to be clear that *I'm not asking you to eat less*. If you're not eating enough at mealtimes to stay satiated for at least three to four hours, then your meals might not be big enough. Today, consider making your meals more satiating and try to minimize snacking as much as possible. Whenever you feel the urge to snack, check out the feeling item below to see if maybe what you're feeling isn't hunger after all.

Feeling: Find Out What You're Feeling

When you slow down and start to live in the present moment, allowing your feelings and emotions to come to the surface, you might struggle to articulate exactly what you are feeling. Emotions aren't as simple as "happy," "sad," "excited," or "angry." After all, we humans are complex beings. One of my favorite tools for identifying different emotions is the Wheel of Emotions, which was created by Dr. Robert Plutchik, a psychologist who wrote or cowrote more than 260 articles and eight books. As you go through the 21-day plan, refer to this wheel to put your finger on exactly what it is that you're feeling. The vast array of emotions you feel every single day might surprise you. But don't worry—that just means you're human.

Gut Feelings

114

DAY 3

Let's Have "The Talk" . . . The Sugar Talk

As we learned in chapter 2, if there's one food that sabotages health and happiness and contributes to Shameflammation more than any other, it's sugar. More specifically, it's added, refined, and unnecessary sugars that somehow find their way into our daily diet. Sugar is hiding everywhere—it's not just in our desserts; it's in our cereal, sauces, yogurts, and even salad dressings. Sugar is also hiding under a bunch of different names—anything from *corn syrup, cane syrup, agave nectar, turbinado,* or *maltodextrin* to anything with suffix *-ose.* Therefore, while our plates might not be loaded with cakes, cookies, or candy, we can still end up consuming a whole lot of sugar from sneaky sources. Today is all about turning our attention to sugar and the role it plays in our lives.

Gut: Do a Sugar Audit

A sugar audit can be accomplished in a few ways. You can simply look at the grams of added sugar in the foods you eat, or if it feels right, you can write them down and tally them up at the end of the day to see how many grams of sugar you think you are typically consuming. Then your task is to reflect on your sugar intake and the most common sources of sugar in your life. Now, I called today's task an audit because I want you to do this in a clinical way. Don't judge yourself, beat yourself up, or make sugar into an enemy. Simply assess the situation. When you have an understanding of your sugar situation, ask yourself which sources of sugar bring you the most joy. For example, maybe you live for your oat milk latte every morning, and that half cup of milk you use has 8 grams of sugar. Or you might love getting ice cream with your partner after a date; this brings you a lot of joy and is a special moment for just the two of you. Those would both be sources of sugar that you should enjoy fully without any guilt or regret.

Inevitably, though, you'll uncover sources of sugar that are less important to your happiness. One great example is yogurt, which can contain a shocking amount of sugar. If you start your day with your beloved latte and yogurt, could you purchase plain yogurt and add fresh or frozen berries (which contain fiber, buffering sugar spikes) for sweetness? Could you replace the soda you drink with a sparkling water or a low-sugar alternative? Ask yourself if there are opportunities to reduce your overall sugar intake that don't make you feel like you're restricting yourself or missing out on any of the fun. If it feels right, I challenge you to try to cut out those sources of sugar for the rest of the 21 days.

Feeling: Fight Sugar Cravings with a Quick Meditation

So many nutrition and lifestyle experts will proclaim, "Sugar is ruining your health!" "Sugar is the devil!" "Avoid sugar at all costs!" without ever telling you how exactly to go about reducing the amount of sugar you eat. And if you've ever tried to cut out sugar, you know that it's not as easy as you might think. We've all read somewhere that sugar is as addictive as cocaine, but that doesn't really mean anything to us until we try to cut sugar out of our life. Sugar interacts with our stress response in a way that temporarily calms our nerves, which means it can become a way of regulating our stress response. If you've ever scarfed down a box of cookies or glugged a can of soda on a particularly bad day, you've already seen this connection in action. If you can relate to this, don't fret—it just means that you're human and that your body and mind are doing what they were designed to do. What I've found most helpful for sugar cravings is a metaphysical meal, which is a nonfood way of nourishing yourself and quelling your cravings. I gave an example of a metaphysical meal on page 102. You can choose to do that 15-minute practice today. Another option is 4-7-8 breathing (see page 94), a mindfulness breathing tool I love to use as a metaphysical meal for sugar cravings because it can be done anywhere, anytime.

Here's exactly what to do:

- Breathe out, emptying the lungs of as much air as you can.
- Breathe in quietly through your nose for a count of 4 seconds.
- Hold the breath for a count of 7 seconds.
- Exhale slowly through the mouth for 8 seconds, pursing your lips to create

some back pressure and a loud breathing sound—the more noise you make, the better.

◆ Repeat this cycle four to five times.

Now, I know that not all sugar cravings are going to be magically cured by this breathing exercise. But it can help you understand just how integral sugar is to your emotional regulation. Sometimes simply bringing that link to the forefront of your mind is enough for you to take a step back and provide your body with what it really needs instead of a quick hit of sugar.

DAY 4

Find Extra Nourishment

Sometimes we get so wrapped up in what's healthy and what's not that we forget that food is one of the best ways to show ourselves some love. We first receive nourishment as a selfless act on the part of our parents, and eventually we take responsibility for our own nourishment. Each and every one of us deserves to be well nourished. Unfortunately, because of busy schedules, budgets, and other challenges, many of us struggle to care for ourselves as well as we'd like. That's why today is all about nourishment—for our gut and our feelings.

Gut: Lean on Broths and Soups

Soups, broths, and stews are one of the easiest, cheapest, and healthiest ways to nourish yourself. Why? Because you can use frozen vegetables and ingredients, which are typically cheaper, and it can all be done in one pot. Soups are easy on your gut, and they're the definition of warm, comforting, and nourishing. If you left this plan with no other tips, making a soup every week and eating it for a meal a day would be a huge win. As a general rule I find that the patients who incorporate more soups and broths on a daily basis tend to restore their gut-feeling connection more rapidly than those who don't. Aim for having 1 to 3 cups of soup or broth a day as your meal or with your meals. You can find some of my favorite soups in the recipe section in chapter 8, but here's a sneak peek into some of the amazing soup and broth recipes I've created for you:

- Creamy Broccoli Soup With Turmeric on page 193
- Kombu Broth on page 190
- Vegan Tom Kha on page 192

Feeling: Hygge It Up

When you think about nourishment, there's a good chance you think about nourishing yourself from within, just as we did in the gut task for today. But you can also nourish yourself from the outside by optimizing your environment. You may have heard about the Danish concept of *hygge*. Pronounced *hew-guh,* hygge is defined as a quality of coziness that brings a feeling of contentment or well-being. It's no coincidence that Scandinavians are rated as some of the happiest people in the world; people have been hygge-ing in Scandinavia for years. Now it's time for you to get in on the action. Staying in is the new going out, the perfect remedy for burnout. Because if you don't find a time to slow down, your body will pick a time for you eventually.

The sensorial, somatic nature of hygge can really anchor you in a present moment, making your life a mindfulness meditation. Light a scented candle. Enjoy the warmth of a hot drink or a fire, or cuddle up under a soft, warm blanket and read a book. You can also just sit in silence. In this way, hygge can be used as an integral part of calming the fight-or-flight nervous system, which makes hygge a great tool to combat Shameflammation. Hygge is about safety, self-care, kindness to yourself, healthy boundaries, and social connection.

DAY 5

Nurture Your Nervous System

As we learned earlier, the key to fending off Shameflammation lies in bringing balance back to our nervous systems. But healing our nervous systems doesn't always have to look like therapy, meditation, or to-do lists. Today I want you to turn your attention to some unconventional ways to nurture your nervous system to get you out of a chronic sympathetic state and into a parasympathetic state. You can do this with a mix of nutritional nourishment and wellness practices that stimulate that all-important vagus nerve, which acts as a leveler for your parasympathetic nervous system and the regulator of the gut-feeling connection.

Gut: Identify Your Favorite Sources of Healthy Fats

Almost all of us are getting too much sugar in our diet, and most of us aren't getting enough healthy fat. This is a problem for our gut-feeling connection, as fatty acids are the building blocks of our nervous system and our cells. Foods with healthy fats include salmon, avocado, extra-virgin olive oil, grass-fed beef, eggs, walnuts, or chia seeds. These all contain anti-inflammatory fatty acids. Now think about the recipes you can make or the meals you can eat that incorporate one of your favorite healthy fats. Sometimes it's as easy as making the mental leap from "I want to eat more healthy fat" to "Here's how I'm going to do it." Making lasting lifestyle changes isn't about setting goals—it's about figuring out how you're going to get there on a realistic and granular level. As James Clear writes in *Atomic Habits*, "Every Olympian wants to win a gold medal. Every candidate wants to get the job. And if successful and unsuccessful people share the same goals, then the goal cannot be what differentiates the winners from the losers. . . . The goal has always been there. It was only when [the British cyclists] implemented a *system* of continuous small improvements that they achieved a different outcome."[1] Once you've identified some of your go-to recipes with healthy fat, you can also try branching out with healthy-fat-rich recipes like the Egg-Salad-Stuffed Cucumber Boats (made with olive oil mayonnaise) on page 166 and the Oven-Steamed Salmon with Citrus Salad on page 175.

Feeling: Get Chilly

While I think we can all agree that chronic psychological stress is hugely bad for our health, there are actually certain types of stress that can be beneficial. This positive type of stress comes when we try new things, challenge our minds and our bodies, and ultimately end up stronger and more resilient, both physically and emotionally. This concept is backed by science; in fact, it's been named *hormesis* by researchers. Essentially, hormesis means that certain acute stressors can help make our bodies more resilient in the long run and can help us get back in the parasympathetic state by stimulating our vagus nerve. High intensity interval training (HIIT), saunas, and fasting are all examples of activities that have a hormetic effect. So today, let's enjoy some stress.

Another great way to practice this type of resilience is through stressing the vagus nerve, which we know controls our gut feeling and other aspects of our nervous system. There are tons of ways to strengthen the vagus nerve, but one interesting way is through cold exposure. Now, of course you can swim in an icy mountain lake or book a cryotherapy session, but the easiest (and cheapest) way to get a little dose of cold in your life is actually in the shower. We often opt for hot showers out of habit, but cold showers are a great way to stimulate the vagus nerve and increase parasympathetic nervous system activity. In fact, studies have shown that cold therapy may help reduce depression and anxiety via vagus nerve stimulation.[2] So the next time you take a shower, experiment with turning the water to cold and letting it run over your body until you start to shiver. Try to stay under the water for at least 60 seconds and repeat the cycle a few times. You can work up to a few minutes. A more advanced approach is to immerse yourself in an ice bath or cold plunge at around 50°F. When I started experimenting with this, starting off low and slow time wise, I noticed a real improvement in my concentration, sleep, and energy levels as well as a decrease in background anxiousness and stress and in aches and pains. Cold showers are one great way to infuse wellness into your everyday life and activate the vagus nerve for more resilience and relaxation throughout your life.

DAY 6

Explore the World of Elixirs and Adaptogens

One of the biggest problems in the modern world is that it's hard to stay rooted in the present. We're constantly interrupted by emails, calls, notifications, and various other pings, dings, and rings. In addition to creating daily boundaries with our phone, we can also find small ways to combat these constant distractions. These can take the form of physical substances that can help root us in the moment and calm our body, and also in practices and rituals that clear away the noise of being alive and give us the gift of a moment of stillness and quiet. Today that's what we're focusing on cultivating.

Gut: Explore the World of Adaptogens

Even if we practice mindfulness and work to put our bodies back in a parasympathetic state, we all need a little extra support sometimes. The effects of chronic stress, trauma, and negative emotions can make it hard to get a handle on our nervous systems with just lifestyle changes alone. This is probably why a family of herbs called *adaptogens* have become so popular over the last few years. Adaptogens are plant medicines—but not just any old plant medicines. Adaptogens are a broad family of herbs and plant medicines that have been used for thousands of years throughout the world. To be labeled an adaptogen, a plant medicine must meet at least three criteria:

1. It must be generally safe (for just about everyone).
2. It must help you handle stress.
3. It must work to balance your hormones.

You may have already heard of some popular adaptogens, like chaga, reishi, or ashwagandha. Well, they all work by bringing balance back to the connection between your brain and your hormones. This includes your hypothalamic-pituitary-adrenal (HPA) axis, hypothalamic-pituitary-thyroid (HPT) axis, and hypothalamic-pituitary-gonadal (HPG) axis. You need all these communication systems working in perfect harmony to support your mood, metabolism, energy levels, immune system, and sex drive. Your HP axis also controls hundreds of pathways that are responsible for inflammation. And because chronic inflammation is linked to many of the common health problems we see today, the medical literature has found adaptogens to have even more fascinating and far-reaching health benefits, such as reducing stress-related fatigue and regenerating brain cells.[3,4] Like the colors of the rainbow or the superhero kids on *Captain Planet and the Planeteers* (where are all my fellow nineties kids?), the inhabitants of the adaptogenic kingdom sometimes work brilliantly by themselves and sometimes cooperate synergistically with other complementary adaptogens. Here are a few that are particularly good at calming the nervous system and nourishing the gut and the brain:

- **Holy Basil (Tulsi):** This is one of my favorite adaptogens. Studies have shown that people who take this Ayurvedic herb regularly feel less anxious, stressed, and depressed.[5]
- **Lion's Mane:** Studies have shown the consumption of this medicinal mushroom can reduce depression and anxiety.[6]
- **Ashwagandha:** Taking ashwagandha has been shown to reduce anxiety by up to 44 percent.[7]

The coolest thing about adaptogens and medicinal mushrooms is that they can be added to your routine and used in recipes with your meals. Tuning in to our senses is one of the best ways to get into the present moment and quiet the mind and nervous system.

You can find adaptogen suggestions sprinkled throughout the recipes—look for the asterisk.

Feeling: Tune In To Your Senses

One of the most effective ways to get present and connect with the world around you is to use your senses. Today I want you to do an exercise. Sit down in a place where you are as free from distractions as possible. Then take a deep breath and try to identify three things you can hear, three things you can feel, and three things you can smell. When you find the items, really focus on them and the qualities they possess. When you focus on, say, the couch you're sitting on, pay attention to the little details, including the coolness or warmness of the fabric, the stitching, and the colors. When you smell your smells, pay attention to whether they are sweet or spicy and whether they change as you inhale.

DAY 7

Tend to Your Gut

A big chunk of what you've learned so far in this book is about how the gut bacteria that make up our microbiome rule our health. So it makes sense that some of the action items will have to do with supporting the gut microbiome. But the microbiome itself isn't the only reason why the belly is the center of our health; in fact, belly breathing can be one of the best ways to access a parasympathetic state.

Gut: Feed Your Gut's Garden

I'm a firm believer that fermented foods and probiotics should be part of almost everyone's daily routine. The good news is that fermented foods are delicious and you don't need to eat a huge amount of them to get the benefits; in fact, just a few forkfuls of sauerkraut, a few spoonfuls of a bacteria-rich coconut yogurt, or a few sips of kombucha or water kefir can inoculate your gut with tasty bacteria. Today it's time to grab the fermented food you purchased and give it a try. Then try to eat some of it every day until you use it up.

Here are some tips about buying fermented foods and probiotics:

- Try buying your fermented foods from the farmers' market if you have one. Locally produced fermented foods are typically cheaper.
- Look for a probiotic with at least 50 billion CFUs, which stands for "colony-forming units" (this is the way we measure bacteria).

If you're making fermented foods at home, check out the Make-It-Your-Own Rice Bowl (Congee) topped with kimchi on page 164 or Curried Lentil Wraps with Coconut-Lime Yogurt Sauce on page 168. These recipes include fermented foods and fiber that will feed your gut garden.

You might be shocked to find that more than your digestion will be improved by incorporating fermented foods; other health issues you may have will start to become less severe as well. Oftentimes I hear this from patients with seasonal allergies, food sensitivities, and anxiety. We know that the gut is the center of health, so no surprise there. If you are new to probiotic-rich foods, start off low and slow to allow your microbiome time to adjust.

Feeling: Breathe into Your Belly

One of the most jarring ways we humans have strayed from how our bodies were originally designed to function is the way we breathe. Let's do a test. Inhale deeply and then hold your breath. Did you feel your shoulders move up or your chest expand? If you did, then I want you to try something else. Sit with your back straight and your shoulders relaxed. Now when you breathe in, send the air down to your belly and allow it to expand. Then when you breathe out, pull your belly in toward your spine. *That* is how you're supposed to breathe. Repeat that five times for some five times a day and you'll be well on your way to a more relaxed body and mind. This might seem painfully simple, but it is a great metaphysical meal. Belly breathing has endless benefits, including relaxing your nervous system and strengthening your vagus nerve, which as we know is one of the main connectors of the brain and gut.

DAY 8

Optimize Your Evening

One of the most underrated health practices—sleep—is key to fending off Shame-flammation. Why? Because it allows our brain time to sort memories and rest from the day, and it is key to processing the emotional experiences that we have throughout the day. Many of us think we can skimp on sleep if we just do enough of the other stuff, but the truth is, no amount of nutrient-dense food or workouts can make up for high-quality z's. Our action items for today involve optimizing sleep.

Gut: Set Up Your Sleep for Success

You might not believe it, but your gut bacteria are intricately involved in regulating your sleep-wake cycle. Don't believe me? Studies have shown that factors like pulling an all-nighter or traveling to a different time zone can cause changes to the gut bacteria that may contribute to weight gain and metabolic conditions.[8] In fact, a fascinating study published in *PLoS One* showed that a species of human gut bacteria called *Enterobacter aerogenes* actually has its own circadian rhythm and responds to fluctuations in the hormone melatonin.[9] Today I want you to think of one way you could make your sleep better. This could include any of the following:

- Reduce your afternoon caffeine consumption.
- Turn off all screens an hour before bed.
- Cover clocks, fans, and any other sources of light in your room and get blackout blinds or curtains.
- Set the temperature of your bedroom to the optimal temperature for sleep, which for adults is between 60 and 67 degrees.
- Go outside first thing in the morning for a few minutes of direct sun exposure. This helps signal to your body that it's morning and sets up your circadian rhythm for success.
- Try taking magnesium glycinate 30 minutes to an hour before bed. It has a calming effect and promotes sleep.
- Eat foods that promote sleep, such as tart cherry juice and turkey.

Feeling: End the Day with Gratitude

When it comes to emotional health, gratitude can't be left out of the conversation. Why? Because gratitude has a long list of benefits, including reduced levels of inflammation and decreased sympathetic activation in the body. One study from

UCLA showed that feelings of thankfulness improve overall health by reducing inflammation and turning down brain activity associated with the stress response.[10] Such feelings resulted in reductions in the activity in the amygdala, which as we know is the brain's fear center and what sets off chronic sympathetic activation.

Research has also found links between gratitude and humility and brain structures tied to social bonding and stress relief. The feeling of gratitude is linked to higher levels of the feel-good chemical that your body makes, called *oxytocin*. Research on gratitude and humility has also found associations with other health benefits, including general well-being, better sleep, more generosity, and less depression. Gratitude and humility are key in our social lives and in our evolution as a species. Gratitude, humility, and kindness are essential oils for the soul. A little goes a long way, elevating your space with just a few drops. Be a proverbial diffuser of these oils.

Having gratitude practice in the evenings might seem unrelated to sleep, but in addition to the long list of benefits mentioned above that gratitude can provide, it can even improve your sleep.[11] If you need some prompts, try this:

- What are five small things that happened today that you can be grateful for?
- Pick one person you interacted with today and explain why you're grateful to have that individual in your life.
- What does gratitude feel like to you in your body and mind? What does it mean to you?

DAY 9

Create More Stability

Many of us have wished for stability our whole lives. Whatever the reason, stability makes us resilient, secure, and confident in our ability to tackle life's many challenges. The good news is that you don't have to wait for outside forces to create more stability in your life. Instead you can cultivate more stability for yourself. Creating more stability for ourselves is the name of the game today, and we'll do that through a combination of focusing on arguably the most stabilizing macronutrient—protein—and a game-changing equation that will give you a more realistic perspective on your fears, worries, and anxieties.

Gut: Up Your Protein Intake

If you take one hot tip about nutrition away from this book, let it be a strong association between protein and stability. Protein helps us build muscle, helps keep us full, and stabilizes our blood sugar. Protein is also key for mental and emotional stability. The amino acid tyrosine, which is found in protein sources like meat and fish, helps your body make DOPA, which then converts to dopamine—your body's main feel-good hormone. Today let's aim to get extra protein through protein-rich foods like cage-free organic eggs, grass-fed beef, wild-caught salmon, and plant-based protein sources like seeds and nuts. If you need some inspiration for protein-rich recipes, check out:

- Chicken with Basil-Anchovy and Broccoli on page 184
- Mushroom-Veggie Frittata on page 163
- Moroccan-Inspired Meatloaf on page 176

Feeling: Balance the Anxiety Equation

If stability makes us feel strong, capable, and calm, anxiety makes us feel pretty much the opposite. If you struggle with anxiety, you don't need me to tell you how unstable it can make you feel—like you're never quite on solid ground or sure about what's around the corner. Anxiety affects most of us at some point in our lives, and many of us struggle with chronic anxiety, panic attacks, or phobias. Luckily, there's a tool that can help us combat our anxiety. It's called the *anxiety equation,* and it goes like this:

Anxiety

=

an overestimation of danger

+

an underestimation of your ability to cope

I don't know about you, but the first time I read this, I experienced a huge aha moment. This really breaks down that terrible combination of consistently overestimating all the things that could possibly go wrong and doing ourselves the disservice of greatly underestimating our own capabilities. So today, let's focus on the last element in the equation. Take a few moments to think about a challenging time you went through or an example of when things didn't go your way. Then think about the strength you displayed and the coping mechanisms that helped you make it through—you're still here, after all. One of my favorite quotes is from a poet named Rupi Kaur, and it goes like this: "and here you are living / despite it all." Understanding our own resilience and ability to cope with life's challenges is a huge part of making sure Shameflammation doesn't rear its ugly head, so today let's make a mental—or physical—list of the hard things you've been through and the things that helped you make it. No human is immune to suffering, but I promise, you're so much stronger than you think.

DAY 10

Mix Up Your Meals

I don't know about you, but I'm a bit of a creature of habit. I love routine, and try to stick to a morning and nighttime routine every day that I can. That said, getting stuck in the same routine can actually be detrimental to your gut health. For many of us, this routine involves eating the same foods day after day and eating while we're distracted. That's why today it's time to mix up our meals.

Gut: Find One New Vegetable (and Learn How to Prepare It)

The key to a diverse bacterial ecosystem in your gut is eating a diverse range of vegetables and other fiber-filled foods. But here's the tricky part: If you're like me, it's easy for you to get into a routine where you eat the same foods for breakfast, lunch, and dinner every single day. So even if those foods are healthy, they might not be supporting gut health as much as they could. The good news is that you can take baby steps toward a more diverse diet. If you want to increase your gut microbial diversity, bringing some new vegetables into your rotation is key. So today, or at least over the next day or two, try a new vegetable and learn how to prepare it in a way that tastes good to you. If you're not sure what to reach for, pick one of the recipes that features less commonly prepared vegetables. I suggest these:

- New Potato and Pea Salad on page 201
- Coconut Collard Greens with Sweet Potatoes on page 200
- Chicken with Artichokes, Asparagus, and Mushrooms on page 180

But feel free to try any veggie. Maybe sauté it in lemon and olive oil, bake it with avocado oil and spices, or slow cook it in an Instant Pot. This will get you out of your comfort zone in the kitchen and strengthen the foundation of your health—the gut.

Feeling: Have a Mindful Meal

Brené Brown once said, "If you don't want to burn out, stop living like you're on fire." Mental and emotional burnout is something I see clinically in my patients at my functional medicine telehealth center almost daily. This provides only more evidence that it's not just about what you eat at mealtime, it's about what you're serving your head and heart. If you're rushing through mealtimes, you're not able to summon all the digestive energy you need to really break down, absorb, and assimilate the nutrients in your food. This can lead to gut health issues and chronic stress. So your task here is to experiment with taking the time to eat a meal with no distractions. That means no TV, no phone, no emailing or work chats. Ideally, you'd be able to take at least 30 minutes to eat, fully chew your food, and create a mindful moment. Take the time to smell your food, examine the colors, notice the textures in your mouth, and chew every last bite. Notice when you start to go from hungry to full and how much more satiated you feel when you take the time to notice your food and appreciate it fully. This isn't about eating less; it's about not letting delicious and satisfying food go unnoticed and uncelebrated!

DAY 11

Soak Up the Sun

◇◇

As much as we like to deny it, we are still creatures of our environment. Well, one of the most fundamental parts of our natural world is the sun. The sun provides us with warmth and with fundamental nutrients that bolster our immune system and mood. We often focus on the negative aspects of sun exposure, which are real and can be dangerous, but today is all about honoring the sun and all that it provides when experienced in safe doses. Today let's reconnect with the sun and allow it to brighten up our day.

Gut: Get Aware of Your Vitamin D

I encourage all my patients to get tested yearly or biannually for vitamin D. It's one of the most common nutrient deficiencies in the world and plays a role in a host of different health issues, from chronic infections to depression to cancer. This can take the form of scheduling a blood test for vitamin D. Ideally, you'd know your starting point before deciding whether you need to supplement and, if so, by how much. In functional medicine, we aim for optimally healthy levels (not just within the lab's reference range), which we consider to be somewhere between 60 and 80 ng/mL, depending on the person.

The popular advice has long been, "Avoid direct exposure to the sun as much as possible," but we're learning that small doses of sunscreen-less sun exposure may actually be healthy. The key words here are *small doses*. And these benefits can extend far beyond our levels of vitamin D. For example, studies have shown that getting small doses of direct sunlight on your face and skin is associated with lower blood pressure, which can benefit stress levels and heart health long term. One study showed that those who were exposed to healthy doses of sunshine, even in the winter, had a fall in systolic blood pressure of 3 millimeters, which doesn't sound like much but could reduce cardiovascular events by about 10 percent.[12] The National Academy of Sciences recently even released a report, published in *JAMA*

Dermatology, that says, "although the harms associated with overexposure outweigh the benefits, the beneficial effects of UVR [ultraviolet radiation] exposure should not be ignored in developing new sun safety guidelines."[13] So that's why today's feeling task is to try to get a little bit of sun directly on your skin. It's possible to enjoy the benefits of the sun while still doing what is necessary to protect your skin and avoid increasing your risk for skin cancer. Now, I am not advocating you stop protecting yourself with sunscreen or throw caution to the wind! I know your next question is "How much sun is enough—and how much is too much?" Here's a useful chart to help gauge what levels of sun exposure are safe for you (a number measured in something called a *standard erythemal dose,* or SED), based on your skin tone and the UV index on any given day:

- Very Fair: 1–2
- Fair: 2–3
- Olive: 4–5
- Moderately Dark: 5–6
- Dark or Very Dark: 7–8

To calculate the sunlight dose that your skin can tolerate without any damage, divide 60 minutes by the UV index to find out how many minutes outdoors it will take for you to get a SED, which is the fixed amount of sunlight it takes to start getting a burn. For example, if the UV index is 7, you divide 60 by 7, which is 8 minutes. If you're olive-toned, you'd multiply 5 (SED) by 8 minutes, which is about 40 minutes—that's the *maximum* amount of time you could be exposed to the sun without risking a burn. Now, I'm not suggesting you get 40 minutes of direct sunlight every day (as I said, we don't want to risk a burn) if you're olive-toned, but I recommend aiming for at least 5 to 10 minutes any day you can. And of course, if you fall into the Very Fair or Fair category, you'll want to be even more careful and aim for just a few minutes a day.

Since it's difficult to get vitamin D exclusively through food and most of us don't spend enough time outside in the sun, supplementation may be necessary. Based on where your starting level is, I typically suggest supplementing with anywhere between 2,000 and 6,000 IU of vitamin D each day. Look for supplements without added fillers or colors, and retest every two or three months to ensure your levels don't go too high (which I'd classify as above 100 ng/mL).

Feeling: Try an Infrared Sauna

If you live in a colder climate and you're not able to get the sun on your skin, a great option for boosting your mood and getting that sweet warmth is an infrared sauna. Saunas have been a healthy tradition for centuries. The first saunas were built in Finland around 2000 BCE and were just pits dug in a slope in the ground and closed off with animal skins, which trapped the heat inside. These saunas became a social and cultural cornerstone. These days, we don't need to rely on a dirty cave carved into a hill. Instead, we have infrared saunas, which use infrared light to penetrate your body's skin barrier to raise your core temperature. This is different from a traditional sauna, in which the air must be heated before it actually heats you. Because of these differences, an infrared sauna gets less hot, allowing you to spend more time inside reaping the benefits.

Infrared saunas typically emit far-infrared, but the infrared spectrum consists of three different wavelengths, each with their own healing capabilities. Near-infrared (NIR) penetrates the least past the skin barrier to help more on a surface level by fighting against signs of aging and helping to heal wounds. Mid-infrared (MIR) goes a little deeper, and far-infrared (FIR) goes the deepest into the body. These days we also know that the benefits of saunas aren't just theoretical; for example, a small study with two participants showed that after twenty days of consistent infrared sauna use, participants with chronic fatigue syndrome saw significant improvement in their symptoms.[14] Other studies have shown that sauna use can promote mental well-being and relaxation. For example, multiple studies have shown that saunas can lower levels of cortisol by as much as 10 to 40 percent.[15]

Saunas are especially helpful if you're not able to exercise due to a health issue, a physical limitation, or an injury. You can use sauna time to incorporate the Four Steps of the Metaphysical Meal: stillness, sweetening judgment, setting intentions, and sealing your meal.

DAY 12

Create Daily Boundaries

Now, these aren't the kind of boundaries you might expect. These boundaries don't involve interpersonal relationships; instead, the boundaries we're working on today involve your daily schedule and the internal boundaries you set with yourself. Keep reading to find out exactly what I mean.

Gut: Leave a Gap Between Dinner and Breakfast

Intermittent fasting has a reputation of being hard-core, overly restrictive, and designed only for extreme biohackers or health nuts. But actually, intermittent fasting can be as easy as leaving a gap between dinner and breakfast the next day, which we do naturally already. To truly get the benefits of intermittent fasting, we can try to extend the number of hours between dinner and breakfast to at least 12 hours. This allows your body to shift into fat-burning mode, helps jump-start repair mechanisms in the body that help fend off disease and keep your cells in tip-top shape, and gives your digestive system a rest. When I'm in the habit of intermittent fasting, I feel more emotionally stable and clearheaded, and my productivity goes through the roof. For today's gut task, try to leave at least 12 hours (but up to as many as 18) between dinner and breakfast. Instead of waking up and eating breakfast first thing, try tea or some black coffee and wait to see when you actually get hungry. This is truly one of the simplest things you can do to improve your gut health, your metabolic health, and your overall health, and it doesn't require you to change a thing about your actual diet or the amount of food you consume. If it feels right, maintain this habit through the rest of the plan. You might just find it becomes a permanent part of your routine. Remember that this doesn't have to feel forced. When you start feeling like you're swimming upstream, stop. This is all about figuring out what is best for your body and your life.

Feeling: Break Up with Your Phone (or at Least Take a Break)

Let me ask you a question: Do you ever feel like you go through your day back on your heels, feeling frazzled and unable to focus on the task at hand? If your answer is yes, all I can say is . . . same. A big part of that is our phones, which have gotten so sophisticated and convenient that we have more content, more distraction, and more information than we could read or watch in a thousand lifetimes right in our hands at all hours of the day. For many of us, our phones act like a drug, eliciting compulsive, addictive behavior. Studies show that smartphones are rewiring our brains, decreasing our memory and attention spans as well as increasing our anxiety. Almost every human on earth has a smartphone within arm's reach nearly all the time. Shockingly, Americans check their phones 96 times a day, meaning once every 10 minutes. In a very short period of time, we have found ourselves all hooked on the same drug, endlessly scrolling through FOMO-inducing content. Think of a couple on a romantic date, but both looking at their phones, or parents enthralled by their screens as their little ones are calling for their attention. Everywhere you look, you will find someone lost in online distraction. Again, just because something is common doesn't make it acceptable. Technology is not all bad, but we must create boundaries with technology each day to stay sane and give our brain some space. Here are some options:

- Put your phone in a basket when you're at home, using it only when you actively need it, and leave it there until you step out the door.
- Put your phone on silent. Check on yourself half as much as you check social media.
- Turn off notifications or put it on airplane mode so you aren't constantly tempted to check your phone. I tell my patients this all the time: Turning off your notifications is a form of self-care.
- Consider keeping your phone free of social media apps or at least limiting them and turning off notifications.
- Unfollow social media accounts that bring you down. Social media can make you feel that you're missing out or not doing enough—you're not cool enough, not popular enough, not loved enough, not included enough, and of course,

not healthy or happy enough. Instead of being sucked in by endless FOMO-inducing content, set healthy boundaries on what you consume for the sake of your mental health. That's why I make my social media feed a safe, positive space and encourage you to do the same.

The goal here is to love yourself so much that you don't need a phone to distract you from being fully present in your body. You'll find healing in the present, sitting in the stillness. If you or those around you think you spend too much time on your phone, I encourage you to go on this digital detox. So disconnect to reconnect. Immerse yourself in conversations with your loved ones; play with your pets more; meditate. Simplify and de-stress your life. Boundaries are medicine, not only with people but with foods that don't love you back and with technology.

DAY 13

Don't Forget Your H20

Water, like sunlight, is a basic human need that we often forget. Water is probably our greatest wellness tool, yet many of us—even the most health conscious—forget to drink enough of it. We also sometimes forget how restorative and healing bathing can be and why as humans we crave being in the water so much. Remember when I said this plan was all about the simple things that have a massive impact? Today is the perfect example of that.

Gut: Track Your Water Intake

You hear all the time about drinking eight 8-ounce glasses of water a day. Many of us hear that number and think to ourselves: *Eh, what I'm doing is close to that . . . at least I think it is!* When it comes to water, try to be a little more accurate than that. Keep a water journal for a few days to see if you're actually drinking as much as you think you are. One great way to drink more water is to simply start your day with a big glass of water. You can even add a squeeze of fresh lemon for an invigorating boost for your cells and senses. It's not just the amount but also the type of water you're drinking. For example, a study found 316 contaminants in U.S. drinking water. A staggering 202 of those contaminants had no safety standards, and an estimated 132 million Americans in forty-five states have unregulated pollutants in their tap water.[16] That's why I recommend taking today to think about the quantity and quality of water you drink. The good news is that there's a great water filter for every budget. Here are some that I recommend.

Clearly Filtered: $

I love the Clearly Filtered pitchers and water bottles. They filter out all the major concerns while being easy on your bank account.

The Berkey Water Filter System or AquaTru: $$

The Berkey Water Filter System and AquaTru are two options for countertop systems that requires little installation.

Reverse Osmosis Home System: $$$

If you are looking for a quality home system, I recommend the Ultimate Series Permeate Pumped Reverse Osmosis Drinking Water Home System.

Feeling: Unwind in the Water

Water isn't just healing when we consume it internally; it can also be a great tool externally as part of a metaphysical meal. The perfect example of this is a bath, which is one of the most underrated wellness practices out there. A hot bath could consist of your running the water, plopping in the tub, and watching Netflix while you soak. And hey, there's nothing wrong with a little bit of Netflix! But as an alternative, why not turn your bath into a metaphysical meal by infusing it with mindfulness. I recommend putting away all technology, turning down the lights (and maybe even using candles), and creating a bath-time ritual that will truly be restorative. The first step includes going beyond just soap and water by adding Epsom salts to your bath. Epsom salts are one of my favorite ways to de-stress and relieve tension. They're also a great way to give your body a much-needed dose of magnesium, which is often referred to as the *relaxation mineral* or *nature's chill pill*. Epsom salts are just magnesium sulfate salts, so they provide many of the same benefits as magnesium, which many of us are deficient in. Deficiencies in magnesium can stress the body and contribute to headaches, anxiety, restlessness, and difficulty sleeping. There are multiple mysterious connections between magnesium and our mental health, which may be explained by the fact that magnesium supports the parasympathetic nervous system and is an important cofactor in the creation of serotonin and dopamine, two neurotransmitters that play a very important role in mood and relaxation.[17] Magnesium also happens to affect GABA, the main inhibitory neurotransmitter in the brain and the target of antianxiety drugs. Studies have also linked low levels of magnesium to an increased risk for mood disorders.[18] The best way to get the benefits of magnesium is to take it internally through a supplement, but some research suggests you may also get some benefits from adding magnesium to your bath in the form of Epsom salts. This is a form of transdermal magnesium therapy that has helped many of my patients with pain and anxiety. I also recommend adding a few drops of lavender or eucalyptus essential oil to the bath, to activate your sense of smell. While you soak, take long, deep breaths and focus on the feeling of the water on your body and the smell of the essential oil. Make your way through the Four Steps of the Metaphysical Meal, and watch your bath transform into a mindfulness ritual. If you don't have a bathtub, you can also do a magnesium foot bath by filling a pot, bucket, or container with warm water and submerging your feet.

SOOTHING BATH RECIPE
- Fill the tub with warm water.
- Add 2 cups Epsom salts and stir the water until fully dissolved.
- Add 5 to 10 drops lavender or eucalyptus essential oil.
- Soak for at least 20 minutes.

DAY 14

Let Love Guide You

One of the consequences of a dysfunctional gut-feeling connection is a loss of love for food. Food should be exciting, pleasurable, and something to celebrate and look forward to. The antidote to this is reigniting that spark of love—love for yourself, love for food, love for life. Today's tasks are all about tuning in to what you love and letting that guide you to better health.

Gut: Get Excited About Food

I often see patients who have spent so long worrying about what to eat and what not to eat that they have lost all excitement and passion for food. This just isn't right. Food is one of the great pleasures of life. That's why today, I want you to try and hone in on one food that you *love* that also makes you feel great. Not only do you enjoy eating it, but also you know that it agrees with your digestive system, raises your energy level, and makes you feel truly nourished. Not sure which foods these are for you? Some common ones I hear are sweet potatoes, avocado, and nut butter. Now, once you have your food identified, think of ways to incorporate it into your life for maximum enjoyment. Look through the recipes in chapter 8 to see if that food is in any recipes, and then plan to try one out! Think of new ways to incorporate that food into your daily routine. If you need some inspiration, check out Crab-Salad-Stuffed Avocados (page 211) and the Chocolate Pudding with Coconut Whipped Cream (page 206); these two recipes bring me massive joy and are examples of how a nutrient-rich, stress-free meal can be intensely satisfying and satiating. I always tell my patients that if eating healthier makes you feel like you're missing out, you're doing it wrong. Stress-free eating can help you feel nourished and satiated, and food should always be a source of excitement and celebration in our lives.

Feeling: Write Yourself a Love Letter

I know a few of you are rolling your eyes at this already, but I'm not joking! Self-love and appreciation should be at the core of every lifestyle change or habit. So why not take a pause in the middle of the Gut-Feeling Plan and come up with a list of things you love about yourself? This can be anything from your dedication to your child to the color of your eyes to the way you support your friends to your amazingly awesome public-speaking skills. If this makes you feel outside your comfort zone, that's what it's all about. For the sake of vulnerability, I'll go first:

- I love the way I've created a safe space for my kids to be silly, vulnerable, and totally themselves.
- I love my introverted personality. The older I get, the more I appreciate the fact that yes, I love people, but I also *love* my alone time. Sitting in silence and researching (Enneagram Type 5 here) for hours constitute my happy place.
- I love how I take risks and put myself out there.

It may be easier to think about past compliments you've received, so you can start there. But eventually I want you to be able to point out the things you love about yourself or that make you special without feeling self-conscious or embarrassed. The relationship you have with yourself will be the longest and most consistent of your life—you may as well make it one of love and admiration.

DAY 15

Boost Your Brain Chemicals

The brain is an incredibly complex web of synapses, pathways, and chemicals. Many people think that what's happening in the brain is separate from what's happening in the body, but the truth is, they're intricately woven together, and you can't really isolate one from the other. This is contrary to how mental health is approached in conventional medicine, which focuses on the "chemical imbalances" that cause various mental health conditions and largely ignores lifestyle factors that can support mental health. So today let's talk about some of the things you can do to boost your brain's happy chemicals.

Gut: Celebrate with Some Carbs (Yes, Really!)

As we learned earlier, carbs aren't the enemy. You don't need to cut out all carbs to live your healthiest life; in fact, carbs have some very real benefits for your body and brain, such as helping produce serotonin and melatonin. This explains why many people feel sad and anxious or have trouble sleeping when they go low-carb. If you're curious about the ins and outs of carbohydrates, check out my book *Intuitive Fasting*, where I teach you all about carbohydrate needs and carb cycling. For today, let's talk about how to eat carbs in a way that will love you back. Healthy carbs are carbs that also contain fiber, antioxidants, and other nutrients that promote health and reduce the blood sugar spike that carbs can cause. Today let's try to identify some delicious and healthy carbs that work in your routine. For a full list of healthy carbs, go back to pages 79 and 80. You can also check out the following recipes:

- Morning Glory Baked Oatmeal on page 162
- Wild Rice Risotto with Sweet Potatoes or Butternut Squash and Sage on page 198
- Cajun Tuna Salad with Chickpeas on page 169

Feeling: Rethink Your Relationship with Tears

Writer and activist Glennon Doyle brilliantly said: "Crying is good. It's organic baptism. It's how we submerge and begin again." Who doesn't like a good cry? I'm talking about the emotional release of crying. Crying may be one of your best mechanisms to self-soothe. Researchers have found that crying activates the parasympathetic nervous system and that trying to repress crying and emotions has been linked to a compromised immune system, cardiovascular disease, hypertension, stress, anxiety, and depression.[19] Crying emotional tears flushes stress hormones out of our system. In fact, researchers have established that crying releases oxytocin and endogenous opioids, also known as endorphins. These feel-good chemicals help ease both physical and emotional pain and are a way that we can self-soothe. Other research has shown crying can reduce inflammation and that "those who cry are able to better manage psychological stress," according to a study published in a journal called *The Ocular Surface.*[20] Crying has such amazing benefits that the Japanese even have a tradition called *rui-katsu*, which literally means "tear-seeking." This practice involves communal events specifically designed for people to come together to cry—yep, that's right! Participants watch emotion-laden content, and together they flush those built-up emotions from their bodies and brains. Now, I'm not saying you have to spend the day sobbing your eyes out, but this is a great day to reconsider your relationship with crying and think of ways to be kinder to yourself and more welcoming to your tears the next time they come. You could also extend this to your family and friend group. Why not get together to watch a tearjerker or a heartfelt documentary and allow yourself to witness one another's emotion? You may feel tempted to hide your tears or turn away, but I encourage you to accept crying for what it is—not something to be embarrassed about or a sign of weakness, but instead something incredibly healing that can make you a happier, more emotionally resilient person.

DAY 16

Stop Swimming Upstream

For many of you, I know that living a healthy lifestyle can feel like you're constantly swimming upstream. You spend so much time following all the advice out there that you forget to tune in to yourself and listen to your own likes and dislikes, wants and needs. Today is all about making things just a little bit easier and reconnecting with your gut feelings.

Gut: Take a Closer Look at "Healthy"

Today's task involves opening up your cabinets and pantries to take a closer look at some of the packaged foods in your routine, especially the ones you think are healthy. I probably don't need to tell you this, but that isn't any guarantee that they actually are. And one of the best ways to make your life easier is to make sure your efforts to eat healthy aren't falling flat. That's why I want you to look in your pantry, especially at the foods you eat regularly, and look out for words like *natural* as well as for packaging that implies the contents are healthy without including any actual details. Why? Because some common foods are only masquerading as healthy, organic, and low in sugar. Here are some specific foods to look out for:

- Salad dressings
- Protein and granola bars
- Protein powders
- Yogurts
- Cereals
- Oatmeal
- Gluten-free packaged foods
- Crackers
- Processed vegan foods
- Nondairy alternatives to dairy products, such as cheeses and yogurts

When you're shopping, look beyond the front label to the nutrition facts on the back. In particular, check the sugar content on the nutrition label and the ingredients listed. Are there words on the list you can't even pronounce? Are there more than a few grams of added sugars per serving? Does the food contain hydrogenated oils? If the answers to these questions are yes, think about exploring other options.

Feeling: If It's Healthy but You Hate It . . .

Let me ask you a question: If you do something because it's healthy, but you hate it the whole time, is it really that healthy? Today I want to give you permission to think about the things that you're doing for your health that you actually genuinely dislike. Keep this to one or two things and ask yourself: *Can I just not do it anymore?* For example, if you hate walking after dinner, could you do a 20-minute dance class instead? If you absolutely hate drinking your morning green smoothie, could you make a veggie-rich omelet instead? It's normal to get stuck in these patterns of forcing ourselves to do things that we've labeled healthy. But if you grunt and groan and spend your day dreading the thing you have to do, I'm not sure it's so healthy anymore. And science would agree with this. One of my favorite examples is a patient who used to race out of the office to change her clothes, hit the gym, and ride the stationary bike there for 45 minutes before taking a bus home. She absolutely dreaded it—every single day. One day she got to the front of the gym and just couldn't go in. Instead, she walked the almost exactly 45 minutes home. She loved it. She called her mom, saw neighborhoods that she hadn't seen, and discovered a new place. She loved people-watching and the relaxing feel of strolling home, just letting her thoughts wander. What a perfect example of someone saying no to what doesn't serve them! This is such a strong move, and if you can make some moves like this in your own life, you'll be better off for it!

DAY 17

Connect with Nature

In chapter 2, we talked about the importance of activating the parasympathetic nervous system and returning the body to a wonderful state of calm. Today we're looking at two ways to do that, and both involve leveraging the innate calming properties of nature.

Gut: Become a Tea Nerd

If you know me, you know that there's nothing I love talking about more than tea. Tea is such an incredible way to connect with nature. If you think about it, it's pretty incredible that the earth provides us with so many incredible tasty ingredients to brew and enjoy. A cup of tea is a perfect opportunity to tend to the gut-feeling connection and make the simple, mundane things a meditation. Just look at some of the awesome benefits associated with these different teas:

STRESS AND ANXIETY
- Chamomile
- Passionflower
- Kava

GUT HEALTH
- Licorice
- Peppermint
- Slippery elm
- Marshmallow root

INFLAMMATION
- Nettle leaf
- Ginger
- Rose hip
- Green/Black/White teas

Today think of ways to incorporate tea into your regular routine. Could you replace one cup of coffee a day with tea? Could you replace the occasional dessert with a cup of chamomile? There are endless ways to fit tea into your life and possibly get some of the health benefits that come with it.

Feeling: Immerse Yourself in Nature

Ralph Waldo Emerson once said, "Adopt the pace of nature: her secret is patience." Whenever I talk to my patients about metaphysical meals, forest bathing is always something I bring up. I've long been fascinated by the research on *shinrin-yoku* (*shinrin* is "forest" in Japanese; *yoku* is "bathing") and how this practice can be used in our everyday life. Because, while forest bathing might sound like something you do on an expensive wellness retreat, it's really just another word for connecting with nature, which is something most of us can do every single day—for free! Forest bathing is about soaking our senses in the sights, sounds, and smells that are so soothing in the natural world, making nature a meditation. By opening our senses, forest bathing bridges the gap between us and the natural world. Aligning yourself with nature is extremely healing.

Intuition, doctors, and studies all tell us that nature can heal us. Studies reveal that nature can lower stress hormones, heart rate, blood pressure, and inflammation levels and can improve plenty of biomarkers for overall human health such as illness recovery and overall happiness. One study published in the United States showed that forest bathing led to more creativity and better problem-solving.[21] Other studies have shown that this practice decreased stress levels and heart rates; led to less pain and depression; increased happiness, health, and well-being; and even improved cognition.[22] Remember when we learned about polyvagal theory and chronic sympathetic activation? Well, forest bathing has a marked effect on the activity of the autonomic nervous system, calming sympathetic activation and putting you in a better mental and physical state. One fascinating study involved a day-long forest bathing session on 155 adults, of which 37 percent had depressive tendencies. After forest bathing, those with depressive tendencies demonstrated significantly greater improvement in mood scores, and many of them had mood scores that resembled those without any depressive tendencies from the beginning.[23]

So what makes nature so healing? The secret may in part lie in something called *phytoncides,* which are antimicrobial organic compounds derived from plants. It's well documented that breathing in phytoncides can increase the number of immune cells in the body, which would explain the results of one study showing how a forest bathing trip led to an increase in natural killer cells (a type of white blood cell that attacks tumor cells and cells infected by viruses) activity.[24] Even more interesting, the data showed that the increase in activity lasted for more than thirty days after the trip. The benefits of forest bathing may also lie in the fact that many of us are lacking in nature exposure in general. Research shows that by 2050, 66 percent of the world's population will likely live in cities, and the average American spends 93 percent of their time indoors.[25] I recommend starting with a walk in the nature area closest to you, whether that be your backyard, a nearby park, or a community garden. Forests are basically wireless chargers for humans.

And here's the great news—you don't need to hike ten miles through the wilderness or camp overnight to take advantage of the calming and healing properties of nature. I simply try to spend some time in nature every single day—even if it's taking a 15-minute walk without my phone, music, or distractions of any kind. You can also bring elements of forest bathing into your home. Try listening to relaxing music that incorporates the sounds of rain, crashing waves, or birds chirping. You can drink fresh herbal teas with fresh mint or ginger or fill your home with plants. I even suggest decorating your house with natural earthy tones like wood, rattan, and linen. Finally, you can use beauty products, cleaning products, and bath products that are infused with real nature scents like eucalyptus, juniper, and spruce.

DAY 18

Get What You Need

Being human requires constant maintenance. We're not eternal machines that you turn on and leave to themselves. Sometimes we malfunction, slow down, or start making strange noises, and we're not really sure what's going on. It's so important to give our bodies and minds what they need in order to function at their best.

Gut: Eat Until You're Satiated

I know, it sounds simple. But it's not! Whether you tend to restrict calories and portion sizes or do the opposite and tend to overeat and end up uncomfortable for hours after a meal, today is the perfect day to experiment with eating until you're satiated. Instead of restricting or overeating, try listening to your body and allowing it to tell you when to start and stop eating. Now, I know that this is complicated and emotional territory for a lot of folks—you may have a history of disordered eating, or you may be in the middle of a weight-loss or a weight-gain journey. If this experiment doesn't feel right, move on. If you think you might be struggling with leptin resistance or your hunger signals are out of whack, try:

- Moroccan-Inspired Lamb Burgers on page 171
- Make-It-Your-Own Black Bean Chili on page 196
- Curried Chicken Salad with Mango and Cashews in Avocados on page 167

I love these recipes on days when I'm feeling ravenous and often recommend them to patients who struggle with constant hunger and cravings.

Feeling: Try a Sacred Nap

As we learned earlier, sleep is key to health and happiness. That's why one of my favorite metaphysical meals is a sacred afternoon nap. This isn't just any old 20 minutes of snoozing on the couch, either. This is a full-blown sacred nap ritual that will infuse your day with some peace and calm. We've been talking a lot in this chapter about how important it is to give your mind some space in order to restore your gut-feeling connection. Well, one great way to give your mind a rest is to quite literally take a rest. Naps are an excellent way to press the reset button on your day and allow yourself some time to recharge. Deep breaths and deep sleep are little love notes to your body. Research shows that naps can improve reaction time, logical reasoning, and mood.[26] In one study, participants who took a midday nap were less impulsive and had a greater tolerance for frustration than people who took a break to watch a documentary.[27] Napping can help us with learning and memory processing, just like a night of sleep. Studies have shown that a nap leads to better cognitive performance than a cup of coffee. Naps as short as 15 minutes can help reduce stress and tension.[28] Even if you just lie down and shut your eyes for 20 minutes, you can ease a racing mind and give yourself a few minutes to breathe.

DAY 19

Keep Things Moving

Physical movement is one of the most important things you can do for your overall health, but movement doesn't just apply to exercise. The movement of your digestive system—and more specifically, your bowel movements—are also a key part of health. Today we're turning our attention to these two types of movement.

Gut: Get Things Moving

Fiber is something so many of us miss, so today we're taking a closer look at this important nutrient. In chapter 5, we learned that fiber is found in high quantities in plant-based foods like fresh fruits and vegetables as well as in seeds, grains, and legumes. As we wind down the 21-Day Gut-Feeling Plan, I'd like you to turn your attention to fiber and think about the best sources of fiber in your regular routine. Then track your fiber intake today to figure out if you're close to hitting the ideal daily dose of fiber:

- **Women:** 21 to 25 grams of fiber a day
- **Men:** 30 to 38 grams of fiber a day

You could easily hit 30 grams of fiber by, for example, consuming a cup of raspberries (8 grams), a cup of lentils (13 grams), and a cup of overnight oats (16.5 grams). Add in a few other fruits and veggies, and you've easily hit your daily fiber goal so that you can have normal bowel movements (one to two "snakes" a day, as I tell my patients).

If you're looking for ways to get more fiber, try the Kale Salad with Pistachio Vinaigrette on page 203 or the Almond Puff Pancake with Maple-Baked Fruit on page 155. These are fiber-rich options that will help keep your digestion moving and provide all the other benefits we know fiber provides, including helping with detoxification, blood sugar balance, and hunger and cravings.

Feeling: Sweat It Out

Exercise is one of the world's best antianxiety and antidepressant drugs. In fact, one study looked at 127 depressed people who hadn't responded to selective serotonin reuptake inhibitors (SSRIs, the most common type of antidepressant medication) and found that exercise helped 30 percent of them get into remission, which is actually a better result than drugs alone.[29] Pretty wild, isn't it? What's even more bonkers is the fact that very few doctors recommend exercise to their patients struggling with their mental health. Even if you don't have a mental health condition, exercise can make you feel lighter, more confident, and optimistic. Today my challenge to you is to get 30 minutes of exercise and then reflect on how you feel in your body and brain before and after. If you're not sure what type of exercise, here are some simple ideas that require zero equipment:

- Walking
- A no-equipment high intensity interval training (HIIT) workout (you can search for these online and find hundreds of results)
- Walking up and down stairs

Before you exercise, on a scale of 1 to 10 (1 being the best and 10 being the worst), rate your level of the following:

- Psychological stress
- Physical tension
- General well-being

Using the same scale (1 being the best and 10 being the worst), write down any physical or psychological symptoms you might be feeling. For example, you might say something like this:

- Anxiety levels: 6
- Headache: 3
- Lower back pain: 5

About an hour after you exercise, go back and rate everything again to see how things have changed. You might be surprised by just how much your scores improve.

DAY 20

Let Your Feelings Guide You

On the very first page of the Introduction (page xi), I talked about the ancient origins of gut feelings. We all have an intuition that's smarter than we know, and so much of this book has been about slowing down to hear what that still-small voice has to say.

Gut: Ditch Diets and Find the Foods That Make You Feel Good

When it comes to healthy eating, I know one thing for sure: No one diet is healthy for everyone. This causes a lot of confusion and frustration for many of my patients and contributes to health issues and stress. The good news is that once we learn to slow down and get back into the present moment, we can turn our attention to what we eat. We live in a busy, chaotic world, but the simple act of slowing down can help us reflect on the foods that do or don't make us feel good. So today take some time after your meal to reflect on how the foods you ate make you feel. Then start keeping a mental or physical record of those foods that make you feel great and those that lower your energy levels and cause gut issues. Pretty soon, you'll naturally gravitate toward the foods that make you feel great and leave the other ones for eating in moderation, often for special occasions only.

Feeling: Focus on the Feeling

In his book *Atomic Habits*, James Clear says that the real secret to achieving your goals is focusing not on the habits themselves, but on what kind of person you want to be. *Do you want to be the kind of person who invests in their fitness? Do you want to be the kind of person who confidently gives a presentation at work? Do you want to be the kind of person who reads every day*? If you focus on who you want to be instead of what you want to do, it becomes way easier to cultivate the habits that get you to that point. Today, take some time to think about the person you want to be and the habits that that person might maintain.

DAY 21

Take Time for Reflection

Congratulations! You made it to the last day of the Gut-Feeling Plan. My hope is that at this point, you're not relieved or exhausted but instead revitalized and inspired to implement some of the things you've learned or tried to include in your regular routine. Today let's take some time to reflect on the last 20 days and find things that really resonated with you.

Gut: What's Your Gut Telling You?

In the past 20 days, we've covered twenty different ways to care for your gut and your mind. So let me ask you this: Which days were your favorite? Give yourself some time to think, and then grab that notebook and write down three gut items that resonated with you. Maybe it's eating less sugar, consuming more protein, or intermittent fasting for fourteen hours on most nights. Maybe it's focusing on more soups and stews, mindful eating, or a toxin-free beauty routine. Whatever feels the least arduous and the most right to you, that's what I want you to try to incorporate into your everyday life. This plan is all about exploration and reflection, so spend today tuning in to your intuition to see what you've learned and what practices could become something you make part of your everyday life.

Feeling: Imagine a True, Beautiful Story

We all have things in our life that we keep around despite knowing that they're not the best for our physical or mental health. Is there a toxic thought or belief that you just can't shake? It might be something you've believed about yourself since you were a kid or some comment that was thrown your way in a moment of anger. Is there a person in your life you know you could create firmer boundaries with? Is there a habit that you keep repeating or a food you keep eating, even though it never makes you feel better? Whatever it is, today's the day to pay attention to how it makes you feel, and maybe even to find another way to look at it. Try to imagine the most authentic and most beautiful version of your life. What would that look like for you? Are there ways that you are playing small? Write that down and pay attention to the way this version of the story feels, not just in your head, but in your body as well.

CHAPTER 8

Meals as Medicine and Meditation— The Recipes

As we learned in chapter 5, the foundations of a stress-free diet are a fun and diverse range of colorful vegetables and fruits, stabilizing fats and proteins, and some complex carbs that will keep you feeling satiated without sending you on a blood sugar roller coaster. The other side of the coin is to be aware of the damaging properties of foods and ingredients like alcohol, refined carbs, and added sugars. That's not to say you should never have these foods, but ideally your daily habits and routine should make it easy for you to eat them only on occasion.

Other than that, you can focus on eating the foods you love, celebrating the diversity of foods on our planet, and nourishing your body, which does so much for you. The recipes in this chapter aim to do just that—they are simple, fresh, and stress-free. These foods should make it easy to fuel yourself with the ingredients and nutrients that promote a healthy gut-feeling connection and help you stay calm and grounded but also energized and inspired to take on your day. In addition to these meals being medicine, you can support your parasympathetic (rest, digest, repair) system by practicing mindful eating. Eat more slowly, chew your food thoroughly, and don't rush your meals. Eliminate distractions, putting down your phone or turning the TV off. By focusing on how the food makes you feel and practicing gratitude for your meal, you will grow your awareness of the foods you love that also love you back. You will also learn to stop eating once you're nourished and satiated.

I'm so proud of the recipes on the following pages; there's so much flexibility and so many opportunities to choose your own adventure. I encourage you to experiment with some of the recipes in this chapter. You never know what might become a weekly or even daily staple!

BREAKFAST

Almond Puff Pancake with Maple-Baked Fruit

Serves 4

PREP: 15 MINUTES
BAKE: 30 MINUTES

FOR THE PANCAKE

¹/₄ cup ghee	4 large eggs
1 cup almond milk	2 tablespoons pure maple syrup
³/₄ cup gluten-free oat flour or gluten-free all-purpose flour	¹/₄ teaspoon fine sea salt

FOR THE BAKED FRUIT

2 cups sliced fresh or frozen no-sugar-added fruit (such as raspberries, cherries, peaches, blueberries, blackberries, pineapple)	2 tablespoons pure maple syrup
	Unsweetened coconut-based yogurt for serving, if desired

1. Preheat the oven to 425°F. For the pancake, place the ghee in a 9-inch round glass pie plate and heat the plate in the oven to melt the ghee. Meanwhile, whisk the milk, flour, eggs, maple syrup, and salt together in a large mixing bowl. Remove the hot pie plate from the oven, carefully pour the batter into the dish (do not stir the batter into the ghee), and carefully return the dish to the oven. Bake the pancake until it's golden and puffed, 15 to 20 minutes.

2. Meanwhile, place the fruit in a second ovenproof dish and toss with 2 tablespoons maple syrup. Bake the fruit along with the pancake until hot and bubbly, about 15 minutes (slightly longer if the fruit is frozen).

3. Immediately slice the pancake into 4 wedges and place on plates. Top with some of the maple-baked fruit and some yogurt, if desired.

Sweet Potato "Toasts" with Avocado

Serves 4

PREP: 25 MINUTES
BAKE: 15 MINUTES
COOK: 5 MINUTES

2 large sweet potatoes

2 tablespoons coconut oil, melted

Fine sea salt and freshly ground black pepper

2 small ripe avocados, halved, pitted, peeled, and thinly sliced

1 tablespoon fresh lemon or lime juice

2 tablespoons olive oil

4 large eggs

ASSORTED TOPPINGS (OPTIONAL; IF USING, CHOOSE ONE SET)

• Smoked salmon, sliced red onion, drained capers, and Everything Bagel Seasoning

• Thinly sliced radishes, thinly sliced ripe mango or fresh pineapple, lime juice, and Tajin seasoning

• Thinly sliced ripe tomatoes, cooked black beans, sliced fresh jalapeños, chopped fresh cilantro, and lime juice

1. Preheat the oven to 425°F. Line a baking sheet with parchment paper. Slice the sweet potatoes lengthwise into "toasts" about $1/2$ inch thick. Arrange sweet potatoes on the baking sheet; brush both sides with melted coconut oil, and season to taste with salt and pepper. Roast the sweet potatoes until tender, about 15 minutes. Remove potatoes from the oven; cover to keep warm.

2. Meanwhile, mash the avocados with the lemon juice and salt and pepper in a small bowl; set aside. In a nonstick skillet, heat the olive oil over medium-high heat. Crack the eggs into the skillet; season with salt and pepper. Cook to desired doneness, about 5 minutes for runny yolks.

3. Spread sweet potato toasts with mashed avocado, top with an egg, and add toppings, if desired.

Broccoli Turkey Sausage Quiche Muffins

Serves 4

PREP: 15 MINUTES
COOK: 40 MINUTES

FOR THE SAUSAGE

1/4 pound ground turkey

1 clove garlic, minced

1/4 teaspoon ground sage

1/4 teaspoon dried thyme leaves

1/4 teaspoon crushed red pepper flakes

1/2 teaspoon fine sea salt

1/2 teaspoon freshly ground black pepper

1 tablespoon olive oil

FOR THE MUFFINS

1 cup chopped cooked broccoli florets

1/2 cup dairy-free cheddar cheese shreds

5 large eggs

1/2 cup nut milk or gluten-free oat milk

1/2 teaspoon fine sea salt

1/2 teaspoon freshly ground black pepper

1. Preheat the oven to 350°F. In a large bowl, mix the turkey, garlic, sage, thyme, crushed red pepper, salt, and black pepper using clean hands. In a nonstick skillet, heat the olive oil over medium-high heat. Add the turkey mixture and cook until the meat is no longer pink, breaking up the sausage into small pieces. Remove from the heat and set aside.

2. For the muffins, line 8 cups of a standard 12-cup muffin tin with foil cupcake liners, and lightly coat each liner with nonstick cooking spray. Divide the cooked sausage, broccoli, and cheese shreds evenly among the prepared cups.

3. In a large glass measuring cup, whisk together the eggs, milk, and salt and pepper. Carefully pour some of the egg mixture into each cup.

4. Bake the quiche muffins until puffed and set in the middle, about 30 minutes. Cool slightly before serving.

Tip: Muffins may be cooled and frozen for up to 1 month. To reheat, remove the foil liner and microwave at high power for 1 to 2 minutes or until heated through.

Patatas Bravas with Scrambled Eggs and Greens

Serves 4

PREP: 30 MINUTES
COOK: 20 MINUTES

FOR THE PATATAS BRAVAS

2 tablespoons olive oil

1 pound russet potatoes, peeled and cut into $^1/_2$-inch cubes

One 14.5-ounce can diced tomatoes, drained

4 cloves garlic, sliced

$^1/_2$ teaspoon ground cumin

$^1/_2$ teaspoon crushed red pepper

8 to 10 dashes hot sauce

Coarse salt

Fresh lemon juice

Chopped fresh cilantro

FOR THE EGGS

8 large eggs

Coarse salt and freshly ground pepper

FOR THE GREENS

2 tablespoons olive oil

$^1/_4$ cup minced red bell pepper

$^1/_4$ cup minced yellow onion

3 cloves garlic, minced

$^1/_2$ teaspoon smoked paprika

$^1/_2$ teaspoon dried oregano leaves

4 cups trimmed collard greens, thinly sliced into ribbons

$^1/_4$ cup water

Coarse salt and freshly ground pepper to taste

1. In a large nonstick skillet, heat the olive oil over medium-high heat. Add the potatoes in a single layer and cook, stirring occasionally, until golden and partially cooked through, about 10 minutes.

2. Meanwhile, pulse the drained tomatoes, garlic, cumin, crushed red pepper, and hot sauce in a food processor just to break up the tomatoes a bit (do not puree). Once the potatoes have browned, add the tomato mixture and stir to combine. Reduce heat to medium-low, and cook just until potatoes are tender. Keep potatoes warm until ready to serve.

3. While the potatoes cook, blend the eggs in a bowl with salt and pepper to taste*; set eggs aside.

4. For the greens, in a second large nonstick skillet, heat the olive oil over medium-high heat. Add the bell pepper, onion, garlic, paprika, and oregano; cook until vegetables are just tender, about 3 minutes. Add the collard greens and water to the skillet and cook, stirring often, until liquid has evaporated and greens are just tender. Season with salt and pepper.

5. Push the greens to one side of the pan. Add the eggs and cook, stirring to form soft curds, until set. Season with salt and black pepper. Drizzle the potatoes with lemon juice and sprinkle with cilantro.

---

* Optional adaptogen: $^1/_2$ teaspoon moringa powder

Huevos Rancheros with
Salsa-Poached Eggs and Black Bean Chili

Serves 4

PREP: 30 MINUTES
COOK: 20 MINUTES

FOR THE SALSA

2 large ripe red
tomatoes, chopped

1 or 2 jalapeños,
seeded, minced

2 cloves garlic, minced

1/4 cup minced red
onion

1/4 cup minced green
onions

1/4 cup chopped fresh
cilantro

2 tablespoons fresh
lime juice

1 teaspoon dried
oregano leaves

1/2 teaspoon fine sea
salt

FOR THE TORTILLAS

8 store-bought
almond flour tortillas

1 cup dairy-free
cheddar cheese shreds

8 large eggs

4 cups Black Bean
Chili (page 196),
warmed

Thinly sliced romaine
lettuce, chopped fresh
cilantro, sliced
jalapeños, sliced
avocado, if desired

1. In a large bowl, stir together all the salsa
ingredients. Chill until ready to use. (May be
made up to 1 day ahead.)

2. For the tortillas, preheat the oven to 350°F.
Arrange the tortillas on a parchment- or foil-
lined baking sheet and sprinkle each with 1/4 cup
cheese shreds. Warm the tortillas in the oven for
8 to 10 minutes to soften the cheese. Reduce
the oven temperature to 200°F to keep the
tortillas warm until you're ready to serve.

3. In a large skillet, heat the salsa over medium-
high heat until it begins to bubble around the
edges. Break each egg into a small ramekin or
bowl and gently add them to the salsa. Reduce
heat to medium, cover the pan, and poach the
eggs to desired doneness, about 3 minutes for
runny yolks.

4. To serve, place 2 tortillas on each serving
plate, then top with about 3/4 cup warmed Black
Bean Chili. Scoop the eggs out of the salsa and
place one on top of each tortilla; spoon
additional poaching salsa on top of or around the
eggs and garnish with lettuce, cilantro,
jalapeños, and/or avocado, if desired.

Breakfast Fried Rice

Serves 4

PREP: 10 MINUTES
COOK: 10 MINUTES

1 tablespoon sesame oil

2 tablespoons extra-virgin olive oil, divided

4 green onions, chopped

1 cup finely chopped broccoli

1/2 cup finely chopped carrot

4 cups cooked day-old brown rice, at room temperature

1/4 cup coconut aminos

1 tablespoon rice vinegar

1 tablespoon sesame seeds, toasted

1/4 teaspoon crushed red pepper

4 large eggs

1. In a large skillet, heat the sesame oil and 1 tablespoon of the olive oil over medium heat. Add the green onions, broccoli, and carrots and cook, stirring often, for 2 minutes. Stir in the rice, coconut aminos, vinegar, sesame seeds, and crushed red pepper.* Cook, stirring often, until rice is heated through and vegetables are just tender, about 5 minutes.

2. Meanwhile, in a large nonstick skillet, heat the remaining 1 tablespoon of olive oil over medium heat. Crack the eggs into the skillet and cook, covered, until the egg whites are cooked through and the yolks are set yet runny, 4 to 5 minutes.

3. Divide fried rice among shallow bowls, top each with a fried egg. Break the yolk over the rice.

---

* Optional adaptogen: 1 teaspoon astragalus root powder

Sweet Potato and Mushroom Pancakes

Serves 4

PREP: 10 MINUTES
COOK: 20 MINUTES

1 large (12 ounce) sweet potato, peeled and shredded

$1/_2$ of a 5-ounce container sliced mushrooms

2 green onions, thinly sliced

4 tablespoons extra-virgin olive oil or coconut oil, divided

2 large eggs

$1/_3$ cup almond flour

1 teaspoon smoked paprika

1 teaspoon coarse salt

$1/_2$ teaspoon black pepper

Nut or plant-based sour cream or plain yogurt (optional)

Fresh berries

1. Preheat oven to 200°F. In a large bowl, combine the sweet potato, mushrooms, and green onions. In a large skillet, heat 2 tablespoons of the oil over medium-high heat. Add the sweet potato mixture and cook, stirring occasionally, until the mushrooms have released their water, 2 to 3 minutes. Remove from the heat and let cool for 5 minutes.

2. In the same bowl, stir together the eggs, almond flour, smoked paprika, salt, and black pepper. Add the cooled sweet potato mixture; stir until well combined. In the same skillet, heat 2 tablespoons of the oil over medium-high heat. In batches, drop the batter by $1/_4$-cup measure into the hot oil and cook until golden brown on the bottom, about 5 minutes. Flip the pancakes and cook until golden brown on the bottom, about 3 minutes more. Transfer cooked pancakes to a baking sheet and keep warm in the oven while cooking remaining pancakes.

3. Serve pancakes with sour cream, if desired, and fresh berries on the side.

Morning Glory Baked Oatmeal

Serves 4 to 6

PREP: 20 MINUTES
BAKE: 40 MINUTES

3 tablespoons melted ghee or coconut oil, plus more for the baking dish

1 large egg

2 tablespoons orange zest

2¹/₂ cups nut or plant-based milk, plus more for serving

¹/₄ cup honey or pure maple syrup

1 teaspoon vanilla extract

1 teaspoon coarse salt

1 to 2 teaspoons ground cinnamon

¹/₂ teaspoon ground cardamom

2 cups gluten-free old-fashioned oats

1 cup grated carrot

1 cup grated apple

¹/₂ cup chopped pecans, walnuts, or pistachios

¹/₄ cup unsweetened coconut (optional)

2 tablespoons ground flaxseed

1. Preheat the oven to 375°F. Grease an 8×8-inch baking dish with ghee.

2. In a large bowl, whisk the egg, orange zest, milk, honey, melted ghee, vanilla, salt, cinnamon, and cardamom.* Add the oats, carrots, apple, pecans, coconut (if using), and flaxseed. Stir to combine. Pour mixture into the prepared baking dish.

3. Bake the oatmeal until golden brown, about 40 minutes. Let stand for 5 minutes before serving. Drizzle servings with additional milk.

* Optional adaptogen: 1 teaspoon maca powder

Mushroom-Veggie Frittata

Serves 4

PREP: 15 MINUTES
BROIL: 1 MINUTE

2 tablespoons extra-virgin olive oil

One 5-ounce package sliced shiitake or button mushrooms

5 green onions, cut into 1-inch pieces

$1/_2$ of a large red bell pepper, finely chopped

2 cloves garlic, minced

8 eggs

$1/_4$ cup plant-based milk

1 teaspoon smoked paprika

$1/_2$ teaspoon lemon zest

2 tablespoons nutritional yeast

$1/_2$ teaspoon coarse salt

$1/_2$ teaspoon coarse black pepper

Chopped fresh leafy herbs, such as basil and/or parsley

1. Preheat the broiler. In a large broiler-proof skillet, heat the oil over medium heat. Add the mushrooms, green onions, and bell pepper. Cook, stirring often, until the mushrooms are tender, 4 to 5 minutes. Add the garlic and cook, stirring, 1 minute.

2. In a medium bowl, whisk together the eggs, milk, smoked paprika, lemon zest, nutritional yeast, salt, and black pepper. Pour eggs into the skillet over the mushroom mixture. Cook over medium heat. As the eggs set, run a spatula around the edge of the skillet, lifting eggs so the uncooked portion flows underneath.

3. Place the skillet under the broiler 4 to 5 inches from the heat. Broil for 1 to 2 minutes or just until top is set and golden brown. Sprinkle with fresh herbs.

Make-It-Your-Own Rice Bowl (Congee)

Serves 2

PREP TIME: 10 MINUTES

COOK TIME: 15 MINUTES

1 tablespoon coconut oil	1 cup cooked white or brown rice
1 tablespoon grated fresh ginger*	4 cups LIQUID
	1 cup PROTEIN
2 teaspoons minced garlic	1 to 2 tablespoons FLAVORING
2 cups VEGETABLES	Fine sea salt and freshly ground black pepper to taste
1 teaspoon SPICES	TOPPINGS

1. Heat the oil in a large pot over medium-high heat. Add the ginger and garlic, VEGETABLES, and SPICES, and cook, stirring frequently, until fragrant, about 2 minutes.

2. Add the rice and LIQUID and simmer, uncovered, for 10 minutes.

3. Stir in the PROTEIN and FLAVORING; bring to a simmer, then season with salt and pepper. Divide congee between two bowls and finish with TOPPINGS.

VEGETABLES (PICK UP TO THREE): thinly sliced fresh mushrooms, frozen peas, shredded carrots, shredded sweet potato, chopped asparagus, broccoli florets, thinly sliced bok choy

SPICES (PICK UP TO THREE): Ground or stick cinnamon, star anise pods, crushed red pepper, curry powder, ground turmeric, ground licorice root

LIQUID (PICK UP TO TWO): chicken broth, beef broth, vegetable broth, Ginger-Galangal Broth (page 191), Kombu Broth (page 190), canned coconut milk

PROTEIN (PICK ONE): cooked shredded chicken or turkey; cooked peeled, deveined wild shrimp; cooked flaked wild salmon; soft- or hard-cooked egg; diced extra-firm tofu

FLAVORING (PICK UP TO TWO): gochujang, chili garlic paste, lemon juice and zest, lime juice and zest, miso paste, coconut aminos, hot sauce

TOPPINGS (PICK UP TO THREE): sliced green onions, fried shallots, toasted sesame seeds, chopped fresh spinach, chopped kimchi, chopped fresh basil, chopped fresh cilantro, chopped fresh holy basil/tulsi, Everything Bagel Seasoning, chia seed, flaxseed

* Or substitute optional adaptogen: galangal

LUNCH

◇◇

Thai-Style Chicken Larb

Serves 4

PREP: 15 MINUTES
COOK: 10 MINUTES

FOR THE LARB

2 tablespoons liquid coconut aminos	Zest of 1 lime
2 tablespoons fresh lime juice	2 tablespoons coconut oil
1 tablespoon honey	$1/4$ cup thinly sliced shallot
2 teaspoons fish sauce	2 tablespoons peeled and grated fresh ginger
1 thinly sliced small Thai chile or $1/2$ a serrano chile, minced (remove the seeds from the serrano if using)	2 garlic cloves, minced
	1 pound ground chicken or turkey (dark meat preferred)

FOR SERVING

16 Bibb lettuce leaves	Fresh holy basil or Thai basil leaves
Fresh mint leaves	Thinly sliced English cucumber
Fresh cilantro sprigs	Lime wedges

1. In a small bowl, stir together the coconut aminos, lime juice, honey, fish sauce chile, and lime zest. Set the sauce aside.

2. In a large nonstick skillet, heat the coconut oil over medium-high heat. Add the shallot, ginger, and garlic; cook just until fragrant, about 30 seconds, then add the ground chicken or turkey. Continue to cook, stirring constantly, just until cooked through and no longer pink, about 5 minutes. Pour off any accumulated liquid. Then add the reserved sauce and cook briefly, stirring the meat to coat.

3. For serving, divide the larb between 4 serving plates. Surround each serving with lettuce leaves, herbs, sliced cucumbers, and lime wedges. Wrap some of the larb in a lettuce leaf with herbs and cucumbers, and drizzle with lime.

Egg-Salad-Stuffed Cucumber Boats

Serves 4

START TO FINISH: 15 MINUTES

³/₄ cup olive oil mayonnaise

¹/₂ cup finely chopped celery

¹/₄ cup finely chopped dill pickles

2 tablespoons minced green onions (white and green parts)

2 tablespoons Dijon mustard

1 tablespoon chopped fresh dill or ¹/₂ teaspoon dried dillweed

2 teaspoons fresh lemon juice

6 large hard-cooked eggs, peeled and chopped

Fine sea salt and freshly ground black pepper

2 English cucumbers

Hot sauce (optional)

1. In a large bowl, stir together the mayonnaise, celery, pickles, onions, mustard, dill, and lemon juice. Add the eggs and gently fold them into the mayonnaise mixture. Season to taste with salt and pepper.

2. Cut the ends off the cucumbers, then cut them in half crosswise to make 4 halves. Slice each half in half lengthwise to make 12 "boats." Using a small spoon, scrape out the seeds to create a trough; spoon some of the egg salad inside each trough. Before serving, season with hot sauce, if desired.

Curried Chicken Salad with Mango and Cashews in Avocados

Serves 4

START TO FINISH: 15 MINUTES

$1/_2$ cup olive oil mayonnaise

2 tablespoons honey

1 tablespoon fresh lime juice

$1/_2$ teaspoon curry powder

$1/_2$ teaspoon grated fresh turmeric or $1/_4$ teaspoon ground turmeric

$1/_2$ teaspoon coarse salt

$1/_4$ teaspoon cayenne pepper

2 cups cooked chopped chicken

1 ripe mango, seeded and diced

$1/_2$ cup finely chopped celery

$1/_2$ cup chopped toasted cashews

$1/_4$ cup thinly sliced green onions (white and green parts)

2 tablespoons chopped fresh cilantro

2 ripe avocados, halved and pitted

1. In a large bowl, whisk together the mayonnaise, honey, lime juice, curry powder, turmeric, salt, and cayenne pepper. Add the chicken, mango, celery, cashews, green onions, and cilantro; fold in gently to coat.

2. Divide the salad among the avocado halves.

Curried Lentil Wraps with Coconut-Lime Yogurt Sauce

Serves 2

PREP: 20 MINUTES
COOK: 30 MINUTES

FOR THE LENTILS

1 tablespoon coconut oil

1/4 cup diced yellow onion

1 teaspoon curry powder

1/2 teaspoon grated fresh turmeric or 1/4 teaspoon ground turmeric

1/2 a jalapeño, seeded and minced

1 1/2 cups Ginger-Galangal Broth (page 191)

1/2 cup chopped tomatoes

1/2 cup cubed red or yellow potatoes

1/4 cup brown lentils

1 bay leaf

1 cup chopped spinach leaves

Fine sea salt to taste

2 egg-based wraps, such as Egglife, warmed

FOR THE YOGURT

1 cup fresh cilantro leaves and stems

1/4 cup sliced green onions

1 tablespoon fresh lime juice

2 teaspoons grated peeled fresh ginger

1 teaspoon honey

1/4 teaspoon ground cumin

Fine sea salt and cayenne pepper to taste

1/2 cup plain coconut-based yogurt

1. In a nonstick skillet, melt the coconut oil over medium-high heat. Add the onion, curry powder, turmeric, and jalapeño and cook, stirring often, until the onion begins to brown, about 7 minutes. Add the broth, tomatoes, potatoes, lentils, and bay leaf. Reduce heat to medium-low and simmer, uncovered, until the lentils are tender, about 25 minutes.

2. In the container of a food processor, combine the cilantro, green onions, lime juice, ginger, honey, cumin, salt, and cayenne. Cover and process until nearly smooth, stopping and scraping the sides as needed. Stir the herb paste into the yogurt; chill until ready to serve.

3. When the lentils are cooked, remove the bay leaf. Remove from heat. Add the spinach and stir until wilted. Season with salt. Divide the lentils between the warmed egg wraps and roll up burrito-style. Cut in half crosswise and serve with the yogurt sauce on the side.

Cajun Tuna Salad with Chickpeas

Serves 4 to 6

START TO FINISH: 15 MINUTES

¹/₂ cup olive oil mayonnaise

¹/₂ cup finely chopped celery

¹/₂ cup finely chopped red bell pepper

¹/₄ cup thinly sliced green onions (white and green parts)

¹/₄ cup chopped fresh flat-leaf parsley

2 tablespoons fresh lemon juice

1 tablespoon Cajun mustard or whole-grain mustard

2 teaspoons store-bought Cajun seasoning blend

Two 5-ounce cans albacore tuna packed in water, drained

One 15-ounce can chickpeas, drained and rinsed

Romaine lettuce leaves

1. In a large bowl, whisk together the mayonnaise, celery, bell pepper, onions, parsley, lemon juice, mustard, and seasoning until combined. Add the drained tuna and chickpeas, stir to coat, and break up the fish into chunks.

2. To serve, scoop the salad into lettuce leaves.

Lentil, Hummus, and Arugula Salad

Serves 4

PREP: 10 MINUTES
COOK: 20 MINUTES

$1/_3$ cup extra-virgin olive oil

2 tablespoons fresh lemon juice

1 teaspoon Dijon mustard

1 small clove garlic, minced

$1/_2$ teaspoon coarse salt

$1/_4$ teaspoon black pepper

1 cup dried green lentils

One 5-ounce package arugula

1 green onion (green part only), thinly sliced

$1/_2$ cup chopped fresh cilantro

2 cups purchased (or homemade) hummus

2 cups shredded chicken (optional)

1. For the vinaigrette, in a small bowl, whisk together the olive oil, lemon juice, mustard, garlic, salt, and black pepper. Set aside.

2. In a large saucepan, cook the lentils in salted boiling water just until tender, 20 to 25 minutes. Drain the lentils and return to an extra-large bowl. While the lentils are warm, add the vinaigrette and stir to coat. Add the arugula, green onion, and cilantro; toss to combine.

3. In each of four shallow bowls, smear $1/_2$ cup hummus. Top with lentil salad and chicken, if using.

Moroccan-Inspired Lamb Burgers

Serves 4

PREP: 10 MINUTES
COOK: 10 MINUTES

$1/_3$ cup olive oil or avocado mayonnaise

1 tablespoon plus $1/_2$ teaspoon ras el hanout

$1/_4$ teaspoon lemon zest

$1/_4$ cup minced shallot

2 cloves garlic, minced

2 tablespoons chopped fresh basil

2 tablespoons chopped fresh mint

1 teaspoon coarse salt

$1^1/_2$ pounds ground lamb

4 tomato slices

Cut-up vegetables, such as cooked beets, carrots, and/or jicama

1. In a small bowl, stir together the mayonnaise, $1/_2$ teaspoon ras el hanout, and lemon zest. Cover and chill until serving.

2. In a large bowl, combine the shallot, garlic, basil, mint, salt, and remaining 1 tablespoon ras el hanout.* Add lamb and gently mix well. Shape into four $1/_2$-inch-thick patties.

3. Grill burgers, uncovered, over medium heat until 160°F, turning once halfway through grilling, 10 to 12 minutes. (Or cook patties on a stovetop grill pan over medium heat.)

4. Serve burgers topped with a tomato slice and seasoned mayonnaise. Serve cut-up vegetables alongside.

---

* Optional adaptogen: 1 teaspoon ginseng

Tempeh Hash

Serves 4

PREP: 30 MINUTES

COOK: 20 MINUTES

Two 8-ounce packages tempeh, cut into bite-size pieces

$1/2$ cup Italian vinaigrette (see Tip)

3 tablespoons olive oil

1 pound small Yukon Gold potatoes, quartered

$3/4$ cup chopped carrots

$1/2$ cup diced red bell pepper

$1/2$ cup diced onion

1 teaspoon lemon zest

1 teaspoon turmeric

1 teaspoon coarse salt

$1/2$ teaspoon cumin seeds, crushed

$3/4$ teaspoon coarse black pepper

$1/2$ teaspoon smoked paprika

2 cups baby greens, such as kale, spinach, or Swiss chard

1. Place a steamer in a large skillet; add water to just below the steamer. Add the tempeh to the steamer and bring the water to boiling. Reduce the heat to medium-low. Cover and steam tempeh for 10 minutes.

2. In a resealable plastic bag, combine the tempeh and vinaigrette. Seal bag and turn to coat. Marinate for 20 to 30 minutes. Drain tempeh and discard marinade.

3. In a large skillet, heat 1 tablespoon of the olive oil. Add the tempeh and cook, stirring occasionally, until cooked through, 6 to 8 minutes.

4. Meanwhile, in an extra-large skillet, heat the remaining 2 tablespoons of the oil over medium-high heat. Add potatoes, carrots, bell pepper, and onion. Sprinkle with lemon zest, turmeric, salt, cumin seeds, black pepper, and smoked paprika. Cook, covered, stirring occasionally, until potatoes are crisp on the outside and tender inside and carrots are tender, about 10 minutes. Add the tempeh; stir to combine. Add the greens and cook, covered, until wilted, about 2 minutes.

Tip: Use purchased Italian vinaigrette or make your own! In a small bowl, whisk together $1/4$ cup extra-virgin olive oil; 2 tablespoons red wine vinegar; 1 tablespoon dried Italian seasoning; 2 teaspoons Dijon mustard; 1 clove garlic, minced; $1/2$ teaspoon coarse salt; $1/4$ teaspoon black pepper.

Mackerel Salad

Serves 4

PREP: 10 MINUTES
COOK: 5 MINUTES

5 tablespoons extra-virgin olive oil, divided

One 15-ounce can chickpeas, rinsed and patted dry

1 teaspoon coarse salt, divided

$1/2$ teaspoon freshly ground black pepper

$1/4$ cup olive oil or avocado mayonnaise

2 tablespoons Dijon mustard

2 tablespoons finely chopped shallot

1 tablespoon fresh lemon juice

Two 5-ounce cans water-packed mackerel, drained and coarsely flaked

5 or 6 red or green endive, halved crosswise, leaves separated

$1/4$ cup finely chopped flat-leaf parsley or 2 tablespoons finely chopped tarragon

1. In a large skillet, heat 3 tablespoons of the olive oil over medium-high heat. Add the chickpeas and cook, stirring often, until crisp and golden brown, 5 to 8 minutes. Sprinkle with $1/2$ teaspoon coarse salt and the black pepper. Let cool.

2. In a medium bowl, stir together the mayonnaise, mustard, shallot, lemon juice, and the remaining $1/2$ teaspoon coarse salt.* Add the mackerel, chickpeas, endive, and parsley. Drizzle with the remaining 2 tablespoons olive oil and toss to combine.

---

*   Optional adaptogen: $1/2$ teaspoon moringa powder

Make-It-Your-Own Mediterranean Salad

Serves 2

START TO FINISH: 30 MINUTES

1/4 cup fresh lemon juice or red wine vinegar

2 tablespoons honey

2 tablespoons minced shallot

2 teaspoons finely chopped fresh oregano

2 teaspoons finely chopped fresh mint

2 teaspoons finely chopped fresh parsley

1 tablespoon Dijon mustard

Coarse salt and freshly ground black pepper

1/4 cup extra-virgin olive oil

4 cups GREENS

11/2 cups PROTEIN

1 cup halved cherry tomatoes

1/2 cup thinly sliced cucumber

1/2 cup diced red or green bell pepper

1/4 cup pitted Kalamata olives, coarsely chopped

1/4 cup chopped toasted pine nuts or walnuts

1. In a small bowl, whisk together the lemon juice, honey, shallot, herbs, mustard, salt, and black pepper until blended. Slowly drizzle in the olive oil, whisking constantly until vinaigrette is emulsified. Set vinaigrette aside.

2. In a large bowl, toss together the GREENS, PROTEIN, tomatoes, cucumber, bell pepper, olives, and pine nuts. Drizzle some of the vinaigrette over the salad and toss to coat, adding more vinaigrette as desired (store leftover vinaigrette in the refrigerator for up to 1 week).

GREENS (PICK UP TO THREE): chopped romaine; arugula leaves; spinach leaves; thinly sliced cabbage; shredded Brussels sprouts; spring salad mix

PROTEIN (PICK UP TO TWO): shredded cooked chicken or turkey; sliced cooked beef or bison steak; cooked peeled, deveined wild shrimp; cooked flaked wild salmon; flaked canned tuna; drained canned chickpeas or black beans; Marinated Lentils (page 199); hard-cooked egg

DINNER

Oven-Steamed Salmon with Citrus Salad

Serves 4

PREP: 25 MINUTES
BAKE: 20 MINUTES

FOR THE SALMON

Four 4- to 6-ounce fresh or frozen wild salmon fillets, skin on, thawed, if frozen

$1/2$ teaspoon fine sea salt

$1/4$ teaspoon freshly ground black pepper

FOR THE SALAD

1 fennel bulb

1 navel orange

1 pink grapefruit

$1/2$ cup extra-virgin olive oil

Fine sea salt and freshly ground black pepper

3 cups arugula

1 cup flat-leaf parsley leaves

$1/2$ cup thinly sliced red onion

1. For the salmon, fill a roasting pan with 1 inch of hot water. Place the pan in the oven, then heat the oven to 325°F. Coat a cooling rack with nonstick cooking spray. (Be sure the rack can sit on top of the roasting pan without touching the water.) Arrange the salmon fillets on the rack, skin side down. Season with salt and black pepper.

2. Set the rack with the fish on top of the roasting pan. Oven-steam the salmon until the fish flakes easily with a fork, 15 to 18 minutes.

3. Meanwhile, for the citrus salad, trim the stalks off the fennel bulb and cut the white bulb in quarters. Thinly slice the bulb using a mandoline (or into slivers with a chef's knife) to make 1 cup sliced fennel. Add the fennel to a large bowl.

4. Cut off both ends of the orange and set the fruit on a cutting board, cut side down. Use a paring knife to trim the peel and white pith from the orange, following the curve of the fruit. Over the large bowl, cut between the membrane to remove the orange segments; place the segments in the bowl with the fennel. Squeeze the membrane to release any juice, then discard the membrane. Repeat with the grapefruit.

5. Add the olive oil, salt, and black pepper to the bowl and whisk to combine (be careful not to break up the citrus segments). Add the arugula, parsley, and onion and toss to coat.

6. Carefully transfer the steamed salmon to a platter and scatter the citrus salad over the fillets. Sprinkle the fish and salad with coarsely ground black pepper.

Moroccan-Inspired Meatloaf

Serves 4

PREP: 30 MINUTES
BAKE: 1 HOUR

1/4 cup olive oil

1/2 cup grated carrot

1/2 cup finely chopped celery

1/2 cup minced yellow onion

1 tablespoon minced garlic

1 tablespoon grated peeled fresh ginger

1 tablespoon ground cumin

2 teaspoons ground coriander

2 teaspoons fine sea salt

1 teaspoon ground cinnamon

1 teaspoon smoked paprika

1/2 teaspoon cayenne pepper

2 large eggs

1/2 cup finely ground gluten-free oats

1/2 cup chopped fresh mint

1/2 cup chopped fresh flat-leaf parsley

1/2 cup chopped fresh cilantro

1 pound lean ground grass-fed beef

1/2 pound ground grass-fed lamb

1/4 cup tomato sauce

1/4 cup purchased harissa paste

2 tablespoons honey

1 tablespoon fresh lemon juice

Mashed potatoes and steamed broccoli (optional)

1. Preheat the oven to 350°F. Coat a 9×5-inch loaf pan with nonstick cooking spray. In a large skillet, heat the olive oil over medium heat. Add the carrot, celery, onion, garlic, ginger, and spices.* Cook, stirring often, until vegetables are softened and fragrant, 3 to 5 minutes. Remove from heat and let cool slightly.

2. In a large bowl, whisk together the eggs, ground oats, and herbs. Add the ground meats and the vegetable mixture and mix with your hands until well blended. Gently pat the meat mixture into the prepared pan.

3. In a small bowl, whisk together the tomato sauce, harissa paste, honey, and lemon juice. Spread the mixture over the top of the meatloaf. Bake the meatloaf until an instant-read thermometer registers 160°F, about 1 hour.

4. Let the meatloaf stand for 10 minutes before removing from the pan and slicing. If desired, serve the meatloaf with mashed potatoes and broccoli.

* Optional adaptogen: 1/2 teaspoon ashwagandha powder

Korean-Inspired Beef Wraps with Kimchi and Ginger-Sesame Mayo

Serves 4

PREP: 25 MINUTES
COOK: 20 MINUTES

FOR THE WRAPS

1 head Bibb lettuce, separated into leaves

1 cup store-bought kimchi, chopped

1 cup thinly sliced English cucumber

Fresh cilantro leaves

Fresh mint leaves

FOR THE MAYO

1 cup olive oil mayonnaise

2 tablespoons fresh lime or lemon juice

2 tablespoons coconut aminos

1 tablespoon minced green onion (white and green parts)

2 teaspoons grated fresh ginger

1 teaspoon sesame oil

FOR THE BEEF

1/4 cup Ginger-Galangal Broth (page 191)

1/4 cup thinly sliced shallots

1 tablespoon honey

3 large cloves garlic, minced

1 pound boneless grass-fed beef flank

steak or top sirloin, trimmed, diced

1 tablespoon gochujang

1 teaspoon coarse salt

1/2 teaspoon five-spice powder

2 tablespoons olive oil

1 tablespoon sesame seeds, toasted

1. For the wraps, prepare the lettuce, kimchi, cucumber, and herbs and arrange on a platter, keeping each element separate. Chill, covered, until ready to serve.

2. For the mayo, in a small bowl, whisk together the mayonnaise, lime juice, coconut aminos, green onion, ginger, and sesame oil. Cover and chill until ready to serve.

3. For the beef, in a small bowl, combine the broth, shallots, honey, and garlic. In a medium bowl, toss together the beef, gochujang, salt, and five-spice powder. In a large skillet, heat the olive oil over medium-high heat. Add the beef and cook, stirring occasionally, until the meat is seared, about 3 minutes. Add the broth mixture and simmer until beef is cooked through and liquid is nearly evaporated, about 3 minutes. Remove from heat and stir in the sesame seeds. Spoon some of the beef mixture into a lettuce leaf and add kimchi, cucumber, and herbs, then drizzle with mayonnaise.

Goji-Chipotle BBQ Salmon Salad with Lime Vinaigrette

Serves 4

PREP: 30 MINUTES
COOK: 20 MINUTES

FOR THE BBQ SAUCE

$1/2$ cup dried goji berries

$1/3$ cup boiling water

2 tablespoons olive oil or avocado oil

$1/2$ cup diced onion

2 garlic cloves, minced

$1/2$ to 1 teaspoon chipotle chili powder

$1/4$ teaspoon ground ginger

Pinch of ground cloves

2 tablespoons organic apple cider vinegar

3 tablespoons honey or pure maple syrup

1 teaspoon Dijon mustard

Fine sea salt

FOR THE SALAD

3 cups arugula, romaine, or fresh spinach leaves

1 cup thinly sliced cucumber

1 medium ripe avocado, pitted, peeled, and diced

$1/2$ cup diced fresh pineapple or mango

$1/2$ cup diced jicama

$1/2$ cup thinly sliced radishes

$1/4$ cup thinly sliced red onion

$1/4$ cup chopped macadamia nuts

3 tablespoons fresh lime juice

1 tablespoon honey or pure maple syrup

3 tablespoons olive oil or avocado oil

FOR THE SALMON

Four 5-ounce fillets fresh or frozen wild salmon, skin on, thawed, if frozen

1 tablespoon olive oil or avocado oil

Fine sea salt and freshly ground black pepper

1. For the BBQ sauce, soak the goji berries in the boiling water in a bowl for 30 minutes. Heat 2 tablespoons of the oil in a small skillet over medium-high heat; add the onion, garlic, and spices, and cook, stirring often, until the onion is softened and beginning to brown slightly, about 5 minutes.

2. Transfer the onion mixture to a blender; add the soaked goji berries and their soaking water, the vinegar, honey, mustard, and sea salt to taste. Puree the mixture until very smooth, adjusting the flavor with additional salt, spices, vinegar, or honey to suit your taste (the sauce should be balanced between tart and sweet). If the sauce seems too thick, thin it out with additional water. Set the sauce aside.

3. For the salad, toss the greens with the cucumber, avocado, pineapple, jicama, radishes, onion, and macadamia nuts in a large bowl. In a small bowl, whisk together the lime juice and honey. While whisking, drizzle in the oil until blended; set the vinaigrette aside.

4. Heat the grill or a grill pan to medium-high heat; coat the grill grates with nonstick cooking spray. Brush the fillets with 1 tablespoon oil and season with salt and pepper. Place the fillets, skin side up, on the grates and grill, covered, for 5 minutes. Carefully turn the fillets over and brush liberally with some of the BBQ sauce. Grill the salmon, skin side down, for another 3 to 4 minutes or until desired doneness is reached. Do not overcook. Remove the fillets from the grill and let rest while you toss the salad.

5. Drizzle the lime vinaigrette over the salad and toss gently to coat. Arrange the salad on a large platter or on serving plates, then top with the grilled fillets. Serve additional BBQ sauce on the side.

Chicken with Artichokes, Asparagus, and Mushrooms

Serves 4

PREP: 30 MINUTES

COOK: 30 MINUTES

4 tablespoons olive oil, divided

2 cups mixed assorted fresh mushrooms, sliced or halved/quartered

1 cup thinly sliced well-washed leeks (white and light green parts only)

8 spears fresh asparagus, trimmed and cut into 2-inch pieces

Four 5-ounce boneless, skinless chicken breast halves

Fine sea salt and freshly ground black pepper

1 cup chicken broth

1 teaspoon arrowroot

2 teaspoons fresh lemon juice or apple cider vinegar

1 teaspoon honey

4 canned artichoke hearts, drained and quartered

2 teaspoons minced fresh tarragon leaves

Quick and Easy Rice Pilaf (page 197) (optional)

1. In a large nonstick skillet, heat 2 tablespoons of olive oil over medium-high heat. Add the mushrooms and cook until browned, stirring occasionally, 5 to 7 minutes. Add leeks and asparagus pieces and cook until the leeks are wilted and the asparagus is tender-crisp, about 3 minutes. Remove vegetables from the skillet and set aside. Wipe out the skillet and return it to the heat.

2. Heat the remaining 2 tablespoons of oil in the skillet; season the chicken breasts with salt and black pepper. Sear the chicken breasts on one side until richly golden, about 4 minutes, and then turn them over and sear on the other side for 3 minutes. Add the broth and reduce the heat to medium. Cook, covered, until an instant-read thermometer registers 165°F, about 8 minutes.

3. Meanwhile, in a small bowl, stir together the arrowroot and 1 tablespoon of water. When the chicken is cooked through, transfer to a plate and cover to keep warm. Bring the remaining liquid in the skillet to simmer, then whisk in the arrowroot mixture. Simmer the sauce until slightly thickened. Add the reserved mushroom mixture, lemon juice, honey, artichoke hearts, and tarragon. Let simmer for 2 minutes.

4. Slice each breast crosswise, fan out on serving plates, and spoon some of the vegetables and sauce on top.

Chicken Hash with Squash and Kale

Serves 4

PREP: 20 MINUTES

COOK: 20 MINUTES

4 cups peeled and seeded butternut squash, cut into large chunks

4 cups stemmed and chopped curly kale

1 pound boneless, skinless chicken thighs, cut into 2-inch chunks

$1/2$ teaspoon fine sea salt

$1/2$ teaspoon freshly ground black pepper

2 tablespoons olive oil

1 cup thinly sliced red onion

1 cup no-sugar-added dried tart cherries

1 tablespoon minced fresh sage or chopped fresh thyme leaves

$1/2$ cup chicken broth

$1/2$ cup pure maple syrup

1 tablespoon Dijon mustard

1 teaspoon fresh lemon juice

1. Fill a large skillet half-full of water and bring to a boil over high heat. Add the squash chunks and boil until nearly cooked through, about 4 minutes. Remove from the heat. Stir in the kale and let the squash and kale stand, uncovered, for 3 minutes; drain the vegetables and set aside.

2. Season the chicken with the salt and black pepper. In the same skillet, heat the olive oil over medium heat and cook the chicken pieces, stirring often, until browned on all sides, about 5 minutes. Add the onion and cook for 2 minutes. Stir in the vegetables, cherries, and sage. Cook for 1 minute.

3. In a small bowl, whisk together the broth, syrup, mustard, and lemon juice. Pour the broth mixture over the hash and simmer until it is reduced by half, about 3 minutes, stirring to coat.

Chickpea Penne Puttanesca with Tuna

Serves 4

PREP: 20 MINUTES
COOK: 20 MINUTES

3 tablespoons olive oil, divided

4 garlic cloves, minced

1 teaspoon anchovy paste or 1 anchovy fillet, minced

1/4 teaspoon crushed red pepper flakes

One 28-ounce can diced tomatoes, undrained

2 tablespoons minced olive-oil-packed sun-dried tomatoes

1 tablespoon honey

1 tablespoon balsamic vinegar

1 pound chickpea penne or other gluten-free pasta shape and flavor

1/4 cup pitted Kalamata olives, coarsely chopped

3 tablespoons chopped fresh flat-leaf parsley

2 tablespoons chopped fresh oregano leaves or 1 teaspoon dried oregano

2 tablespoons drained capers

Fine sea salt and freshly ground black pepper to taste

Two 5-ounce cans albacore tuna packed in olive oil, drained and flaked into large chunks

1. In a large skillet, heat 2 tablespoons olive oil over medium-high heat. Add the garlic, anchovy paste, and pepper flakes and cook, stirring, until fragrant, about 30 seconds. Add the diced tomatoes, sun-dried tomatoes, honey, and vinegar. Simmer sauce to reduce slightly, about 10 minutes.

2. While the sauce simmers, cook the pasta in boiling water as directed on the package. When al dente, remove and reserve 1/4 cup of the cooking water, then drain the pasta. Transfer the penne to a bowl and toss with the remaining 1 tablespoon of the olive oil. Set pasta aside and keep warm.

3. Stir the olives, herbs, and capers into the sauce. Add the cooked penne and, if needed, some of the reserved cooking water to easily and evenly coat the pasta with sauce. Season with salt and pepper and serve immediately. Top each serving with chunks of tuna.

Steak Diane

Serves 4

PREP: 20 MINUTES
COOK: 10 MINUTES

Two 12-ounce boneless beef rib eye steaks

4 teaspoons coconut aminos, divided

$1/_2$ cup beef broth

1 tablespoon Dijon mustard

2 tablespoons ghee, divided

3 tablespoons minced shallots

1 tablespoon chopped fresh parsley

1 teaspoon fresh lemon juice

$1/_4$ teaspoon fine sea salt

$1/_4$ teaspoon freshly ground black pepper

Prepared mashed potatoes or sweet potatoes

Roasted Brussels sprouts (optional)

1. Trim the steaks of any large chunks of fat and gristle, then cut the steaks into quarters to make eight chunks. Place a chunk in a small resealable plastic bag (don't seal the bag) and gently pound the meat out with a meat mallet to flatten to $1/_4$ inch thick. Transfer beef to a plate and repeat with remaining steak pieces. Rub each piece of beef with $1/_2$ teaspoon of the coconut aminos and set aside.

2. Whisk the broth and mustard together in a small bowl; set aside. In a large skillet, heat 1 tablespoon of the ghee over high heat. Add 4 of the prepared steaks and sear for 1 minute on each side, or until beginning to brown; transfer the steaks to a platter. Sear the remaining steaks in the remaining tablespoon of ghee in the same manner and remove from the skillet.

3. In the same skillet, reduce the heat to medium-high. Add the shallots and cook for 1 minute, stirring constantly. Then deglaze the skillet with the broth mixture, stirring to scrape up any browned bits in the bottom. Return the steaks and any accumulated juices to the skillet and simmer for 1 minute, turning steaks to coat once or twice. Add the parsley, lemon juice, salt, and black pepper and stir to combine.

4. Arrange two steak pieces on a mound of mashed potatoes or sweet potatoes, then drizzle additional sauce on top. Serve with roasted Brussels sprouts, if desired.

Chicken with Basil-Anchovy and Broccoli

Serves 4

PREP: 10 MINUTES
COOK: 5 MINUTES
BAKE: 15 MINUTES

1 to 1¼ pounds boneless, skin-on chicken thighs

½ teaspoon coarse salt

½ teaspoon coarse black pepper

1 tablespoon extra-virgin olive oil

2 cups broccoli florets

2 garlic cloves, thinly sliced

½ cup chicken broth

2 anchovies, minced

1 tablespoon capers

1 tablespoon ghee

1 teaspoon fresh lemon juice

½ cup lightly packed fresh basil, cut into ribbons

1. Preheat the oven to 400°F. Season the chicken with salt and black pepper. In an extra-large oven-safe skillet, heat the olive oil over medium-high heat. Add the chicken, skin side down, and sauté until browned, about 3 minutes. Turn the chicken and add the broccoli florets.

2. Transfer the skillet to the oven. Bake until an instant-read thermometer registers 170°F and the broccoli is tender, 15 to 18 minutes. Transfer the chicken to a serving platter and cover to keep warm.

3. In the same skillet, cook the garlic over medium-high heat for 30 seconds (do not let it burn or it will be bitter). Add the broth, anchovies, and capers. Cook, scraping up any browned bits from the bottom of the skillet, until the sauce has reduced by half, 1 to 2 minutes. Remove from heat and stir in the ghee and lemon juice. Add the basil and stir to combine. Pour the sauce over the chicken.

Ginger-Coconut Fish Soup

Serves 4

PREP: 10 MINUTES
COOK: 15 MINUTES

1 pound halibut fillets, cut into large pieces

1 teaspoon five-spice powder

1 teaspoon coarse salt, divided

2 tablespoons extra-virgin olive oil

One 10-ounce bag frozen mirepoix blend

1 medium (8-ounce) sweet potato, peeled and diced

$1/_2$-inch piece fresh ginger, peeled and grated

2 cloves garlic, minced

$1/_2$ teaspoon turmeric

4 cups vegetable broth*

1 cup stirred unsweetened coconut milk

$1/_2$ teaspoon lemon zest

$1/_4$ cup chopped fresh basil or holy basil

1. Season the halibut on both sides with the five-spice powder and $1/_2$ teaspoon of the salt. Cut the halibut into large pieces. Refrigerate until needed.

2. In a large pot, heat the olive oil over medium-high heat. Add the mirepoix blend, sweet potato, ginger, garlic, $1/_2$ teaspoon turmeric, and remaining $1/_2$ teaspoon salt. Cook, stirring often, until fragrant, 3 to 5 minutes. Add the broth and bring to a boil. Reduce the heat to simmer, and cook, covered, until the vegetables are just tender, 8 to 10 minutes more.

3. Add the fish and cook until opaque, 3 to 4 minutes. Stir in the coconut milk and lemon zest. Cook until heated through, 1 to 2 minutes. Top servings with fresh basil.

---

* Or substitute with optional adaptogens: Ginger-Galangal Broth (page 191) or Kombu Broth (page 190)

Scallop Noodle Bowls

Serves 4

PREP: 10 MINUTES
COOK: 10 MINUTES

12 ounces gluten-free spaghetti or other thin gluten-free pasta

1/2 cup olive oil

2 cloves garlic, minced

3 pints cherry tomatoes

1 teaspoon coarse salt

1/2 teaspoon freshly ground black pepper

1/2 teaspoon honey

1 cup lightly packed baby spinach

1 to 1 1/2 pounds large fresh or frozen sea scallops (about 12), thawed, if frozen

1 tablespoon smoked paprika

1 teaspoon coarse salt

1/2 teaspoon black pepper

2 tablespoons extra-virgin olive oil or melted ghee

1 tablespoon finely chopped fresh chives

1. Cook the pasta in a large pot of salted boiling water until al dente. Drain and transfer to a large bowl.

2. Meanwhile, in a large heavy skillet, heat the oil over medium-high heat. Add the garlic, tomatoes, salt, and black pepper. Cook, stirring often, until the tomatoes burst, 5 to 8 minutes. Stir in the honey and spinach. Let stand until spinach wilts slightly. Toss the pasta with the sauce. Cover to keep warm.

3. Rinse the scallops and pat dry. In a small bowl, stir together the smoked paprika, salt, and black pepper. Sprinkle the scallops with the seasoning. In a large skillet, heat 1 tablespoon of the olive oil over medium-high heat. Add the scallops; cook for 4 to 5 minutes or until browned and opaque, turning once halfway through cooking.

4. Divide the pasta among shallow bowls; top with the scallops and sprinkle with chives.

Thai-Style Chicken Stir-Fry

Serves 4

PREP: 10 MINUTES
COOK: 15 MINUTES

3 tablespoons coconut oil or extra-virgin olive oil

1 pound boneless, skinless chicken breast halves or chicken thighs, cut into 2-inch strips

1 teaspoon coarse salt

$3/_4$ teaspoon black pepper

1 medium red onion, halved lengthwise and sliced

1 red bell pepper, cut into bite-size strips

One 8-ounce package sliced fresh button mushrooms

2 baby bok choy, sliced

$3/_4$ cup diced pineapple

1 tablespoon minced fresh ginger

1 stalk fresh lemongrass, trimmed and minced

3 cloves garlic, minced

1 Thai chile, seeded and finely chopped, or $1/_2$ teaspoon crushed red pepper (optional)

$1/_2$ cup chopped fresh basil

$1/_2$ cup chopped fresh cilantro

Lime wedges

1. In an extra-large skillet, heat 1 tablespoon of the coconut oil over medium-high heat. Add half of the chicken; season with $1/_4$ teaspoon of the salt and $1/_4$ teaspoon of the black pepper. Cook, stirring often, until cooked through, 4 to 5 minutes. Transfer chicken to a bowl. Repeat with another 1 tablespoon oil, $1/_4$ teaspoon salt, $1/_4$ teaspoon black pepper, and the remaining chicken. Transfer chicken to the bowl; cover to keep warm.

2. In the same skillet, add the remaining 1 tablespoon oil. Add the onion and bell pepper; cook, stirring often, 2 minutes. Add mushrooms; cook, stirring often, until mushrooms begin to brown, about 5 minutes. Add the bok choy, pineapple, remaining $1/_2$ teaspoon salt, ginger, lemongrass, garlic, and Thai chile, if using. Cook, stirring often, 2 minutes. Return the chicken to the skillet and cook until heated through, about 2 minutes. Remove from the heat. Top with fresh herbs. Serve with lime wedges.

Beef-Poblano Cabbage Tacos

Serves 4

PREP: 10 MINUTES
COOK: 15 MINUTES

1 tablespoon extra-virgin olive oil

2 poblano chiles, seeded if desired, and chopped

$^1/_2$ cup chopped onion

3 cloves garlic, minced

1 pound grass-fed ground beef

$^1/_2$ cup finely chopped beef heart

1 tablespoon chili powder

2 teaspoons ground cumin

1 teaspoon smoked paprika

1 teaspoon coarse salt

$^1/_2$ teaspoon black pepper

One 8-ounce can tomato sauce

12 medium to large cabbage leaves

One avocado, peeled, seeded, and chopped

Plant-based sour cream (such as Forager brand)

Fresh cilantro

Lime wedges

1. In a large skillet, heat the oil over medium-high heat. Add the poblanos, onion, and garlic. Cook, stirring frequently, until the onion is softened, 2 to 3 minutes. Add the ground beef and beef heart, chili powder, cumin, paprika, salt, and black pepper. Cook, stirring to break up the meat, until cooked through, 8 to 10 minutes. Stir in the tomato sauce and simmer, uncovered, until heated through, about 5 minutes.

2. Spoon beef filling into cabbage leaves. Top with avocado, sour cream, and cilantro. Serve with lime wedges.

Jarred Spicy Ramen Noodles with Tofu and Kimchi

Makes 2 servings

PREP: 20 MINUTES
COOK: 4 MINUTES

4 ounces black, brown, or white rice ramen noodles

4 teaspoons minced garlic

4 teaspoons gochujang or crushed red pepper

4 teaspoons tahini

1 tablespoon unseasoned rice vinegar

1 tablespoon honey

2 teaspoons coconut aminos

1 cup chopped kimchi

$1/2$ cup shredded carrots

$1/2$ cup mung bean sprouts

$1/2$ cup thinly sliced shiitake mushrooms

4 ounces extra-firm tofu, cubed

1 teaspoon toasted sesame seeds

2 cups very hot Kombu Broth (page 190)

2 soft- or hard-cooked eggs (optional)

1. Cook noodles according to package directions except shorten cooking time by 1 minute. Drain and rinse with cold water, then divide the noodles between two $1^1/2$-quart wide-mouth Mason jars.

2. Divide the remaining ingredients* (except for the broth) between the jars, layering each on top of the other. Secure the lid on each jar and refrigerate for up to 2 days.

3. When ready to serve, pour 1 cup of the hot broth into each jar, secure the lid, and shake the jar gently to mix the contents. Remove the lid and microwave the jar in 1-minute intervals until very hot. Pour the jars into serving bowls and top with an egg, if desired.

---

* Optional adaptogen: $1/2$ teaspoon moringa powder

Kombu Broth

Makes about 6 cups

PREP: 5 MINUTES PLUS SOAKING
COOK: 5 MINUTES

Three 2-inch-square pieces dried kombu, wiped with a damp towel

$^1/_2$ cup dried whole shiitake mushrooms

1. Fill a large saucepan with 6 cups water and add the kombu. Let stand for at least eight hours or overnight.

2. After soaking, bring the water to a simmer over high heat. Just before the water comes to a full boil, remove the kombu. Add the mushrooms and reduce the heat to medium; simmer for 1 minute, then remove the pan from the heat and let the mushrooms steep for 5 minutes.

3. Strain the broth through a fine-mesh strainer (save the mushrooms to use in another recipe). Store for up to 3 days in the refrigerator or freeze for up to 1 month.

Ginger-Galangal Broth

Makes 2 quarts
PREP: 10 MINUTES
COOK: 10 MINUTES
STAND: 20 MINUTES

2 quarts vegetable broth

1 lime

2 stalks lemongrass, trimmed

One 1-inch piece galangal root, sliced

One 1-inch piece fresh ginger, sliced

2 green onions, sliced

1 teaspoon coarse salt

1. In a large pot, heat the broth over medium-high heat. Using a vegetable peeler, remove the peel from the lime, avoiding the white pith. (Reserve the lime flesh for another use.) Add the lime peel, lemongrass, galangal, ginger, green onions, and salt to the pot. Bring to a boil; reduce the heat and simmer, covered, for 10 minutes.

2. Remove from the heat and let stand for 20 minutes. Carefully strain the solids.

3. This broth can be enjoyed immediately on its own, topped with fresh cilantro, or stored in pint jars in the refrigerator for up to 1 week, or in the freezer for up to 6 months.

Vegan Tom Kha

Serves 4

PREP: 10 MINUTES
COOK: 20 MINUTES

2 tablespoons coconut oil or extra-virgin olive oil

1/2 cup chopped yellow onion

2 cloves garlic, minced

3 cups Ginger-Galangal Broth (page 191) or vegetable broth

One 13.66-ounce can full-fat coconut milk

1 cup coarsely grated carrots

1 cup sliced shiitake mushrooms or button mushrooms

2 tablespoons coconut aminos

1 tablespoon peeled and grated fresh ginger

1 teaspoon lemon zest

1 teaspoon coarse salt

1/2 teaspoon black pepper

1/4 teaspoon cayenne pepper (optional)

Fresh chopped cilantro and/or basil

Lime wedges

1. In a large pot, heat the coconut oil over medium heat. Add the onion and garlic and cook, stirring often, until the onion is softened, 3 to 4 minutes. Add the broth, coconut milk, carrots, mushrooms, coconut aminos, ginger, lemon zest, salt, black pepper, and cayenne pepper. Bring to a boil; reduce the heat and simmer, covered, for 15 minutes.

2. Top servings with cilantro and serve with lime wedges.

Creamy Broccoli Soup with Turmeric

Serves 4

PREP: 20 MINUTES
COOK: 20 MINUTES

4 tablespoons olive oil or coconut oil

2 shallots, very thinly sliced into rings

1 large yellow onion, chopped

5 garlic cloves, coarsely chopped

$1/2$ teaspoon cumin seeds

$1/2$ teaspoon coriander seeds

$1/2$ teaspoon ground turmeric

1 medium Yukon Gold potato, peeled and chopped

5 cups chicken bone broth, homemade (page 194) or store-bought

$1 1/2$ teaspoons coconut aminos

1 teaspoon coarse salt

Freshly ground black pepper

$1 1/2$ pounds fresh broccoli, trimmed and chopped

1 teaspoon lemon zest

1 (5-ounce) container fresh spinach

$1/2$ cup unsalted roasted cashews, chopped

Fresh parsley, mint, and/or cilantro, chopped

1. In a large pot, heat 1 tablespoon of the oil over medium heat. Add the shallots and cook, stirring often, until browned and crispy, 3 to 4 minutes. Transfer to a small bowl and set aside.

2. Add the remaining 3 tablespoons oil to the pot. Add the onion and cook, stirring often, until softened and beginning to brown, 4 to 5 minutes. Add the garlic, cumin seeds, coriander seeds, and turmeric and cook, stirring often, until fragrant, 1 minute. Add the potato, broth, coconut aminos, salt, and pepper; stir to combine. Bring to a boil, reduce the heat, and simmer, covered, until the potato is almost tender, 8 to 10 minutes. Add the broccoli. Cook, covered, until the potato is tender and the broccoli is bright green, 3 to 4 minutes. Stir in the lemon zest.

3. Add the spinach to the pot and cook just until wilted, about 1 minute. Remove from the heat. Use an immersion blender to puree until smooth. (Or, working in batches, carefully puree in a blender.)

4. Top servings with the crispy shallots, cashews, and fresh herbs.

Simple Bone Broth

Makes about 4 quarts (depending on how much water is added)

CHOOSE ONE FOR YOUR BONES:

1 whole organic chicken or chicken carcass/
bones

1 small whole organic turkey, turkey breast, or
turkey carcass/bones

3 to 5 pounds grass-fed beef bones

1 pound fish bones, shrimp shells, or other
crustacean shells (mussels, clams, crabs, etc.)

Vegetables and Aromatics

6 garlic cloves

1 medium onion, any kind

2 large carrots, scrubbed and chopped

3 or 4 celery stalks, chopped

1-inch piece of ginger, peeled and sliced into
coins

¼ cup apple cider vinegar

1 teaspoon ground turmeric or 1 (3-inch) piece
of turmeric root

1 tablespoon chopped fresh parsley

1 teaspoon pink Himalayan salt

1. Rinse the bones and place them in a large soup pot or Dutch oven, slow cooker, or pressure cooker. Fill the pot three-quarters full with water (or up to the maximum fill line) and add the vegetables and aromatics. Follow these instructions, according to your cooking method:

- On a stovetop, cook over medium-high heat until bubbling, then reduce the heat to low and allow to simmer, covered, for at least 8 hours, adding more water as needed to keep the bones mostly covered.

- In a slow cooker, set on low and cook for at least 8 hours, but no more than 10 hours.

- In a pressure cooker, follow the manufacturer's instructions for broth or soup.

2. After cooking, allow the broth to cool, then strain it through a fine-mesh strainer into a large bowl. Transfer to Mason jars to store in the fridge, or freezer-safe containers for longer-term storage.

Orange and Ginger Beef and Asparagus Bowl

Makes 4 servings

PREP: 10 MINUTES
COOK: 10 MINUTES

2 medium oranges

2 tablespoons extra-virgin olive oil

1 pound boneless beef sirloin steak, cut into bite-size strips (see Tip)

1 pound fresh asparagus, trimmed and cut into 2-inch pieces

One 8-ounce package shiitake mushrooms, sliced

1 small yellow onion, sliced

2 teaspoons peeled grated fresh ginger

2 cloves garlic, minced

1 teaspoon coarse salt

$1/2$ teaspoon coarse black pepper

$1/2$ teaspoon five-spice powder

2 teaspoons arrowroot powder

$1/2$ cup sliced almonds, toasted

1. Remove 1 teaspoon zest and $2/3$ cup juice from the oranges. Set aside.

2. In an extra-large skillet, heat 1 tablespoon of the olive oil over high heat. Add the beef and cook, stirring, until desired doneness, about 3 minutes. Transfer beef to a bowl and cover to keep warm.

3. Add the remaining oil to the skillet and reduce the heat to medium-high. Add the asparagus, mushrooms, and onion. Cook, stirring, until the asparagus is crisp-tender, about 4 minutes. Add the ginger and garlic and cook, stirring, for 1 minute.

4. Return the beef to the skillet. Add the salt, black pepper, and five-spice powder, and stir to combine. In a small bowl, stir together the orange zest and juice and arrowroot powder until smooth. Stir into the beef mixture and cook over medium heat until the sauce is slightly thickened, 1 to 2 minutes. Sprinkle servings with almonds.

Tip: Freeze the steak for 20 minutes before slicing to make the job easier.

Make-It-Your-Own Black Bean Chili

Serves 8

PREP: 30 MINUTES
COOK: 30 MINUTES

1/4 cup extra-virgin olive oil

2 tablespoons whole cumin seed

2 tablespoons dried oregano leaves

2 cups diced yellow onion

2 cups VEGETABLES

1 1/2 cups diced red and/or green bell pepper

1 tablespoon minced garlic

1 jalapeño, seeded and minced

2 teaspoons smoked paprika

1/2 teaspoon cayenne pepper

One 28-ounce can diced tomatoes, undrained

4 cups cooked black beans (if using canned, drain and rinse beans)

2 cups PROTEIN

1 cup LIQUID (if needed)

1 tablespoon fresh lime juice or organic apple cider vinegar

Coarse salt

TOPPINGS

1. Heat the oil in a large pot over medium-high heat. Add the cumin, oregano, and onion and cook, stirring frequently, until the onion is soft, about 5 minutes. Add the VEGETABLES, bell pepper, garlic, jalapeño, paprika, and cayenne and cook, stirring frequently, until the vegetables are soft and garlic is fragrant, about 5 minutes.

2. Add the tomatoes and black beans and simmer, uncovered, for 10 minutes.

3. Stir in the PROTEIN and LIQUID (if needed); bring to a simmer, then season with lime juice and salt. Finish with TOPPINGS.

VEGETABLES (PICK UP TO TWO): cubed sweet potato, cubed butternut squash, sliced mushrooms

PROTEIN (PICK ONE): shredded cooked chicken; cubed cooked beef or bison steak; cooked peeled, deveined wild shrimp

LIQUID (PICK ONE): vegetable broth, chicken broth, beef broth

TOPPINGS (PICK UP TO THREE): sliced jalapeños, plant-based cheddar cheese shreds, chopped fresh cilantro, sliced green onions, diced avocado

SIDES

Quick and Easy Rice Pilaf

Serves 4

PREP: 10 MINUTES
COOK: 3 MINUTES
BAKE: 30 MINUTES

3 tablespoons ghee, coconut oil, or olive oil

$1/_4$ cup minced shallots

1 garlic clove, minced

$1/_2$ teaspoon dried thyme leaves

$1/_2$ teaspoon fine sea salt

1 cup long-grain brown rice

2 cups chicken broth, vegetable broth, Kombu Broth (page 190), or Ginger-Galangal Broth (page 191)

Chopped fresh thyme or flat-leaf parsley (optional)

1. Preheat the oven to 425°F. In an ovenproof saucepan, heat the ghee over medium-high heat. Add the shallots, garlic, thyme, and salt. Cook, stirring often, until shallot is tender, about 3 minutes.

2. Add the rice and stir to coat with the fat, toasting the grains lightly. Add the broth and bring to a simmer.

3. Cover the pan with a tight-fitting lid and transfer it to the oven. Bake the rice until the liquid has evaporated and the rice is tender, 30 to 40 minutes. Let stand, covered, for 5 minutes before stirring in the herbs, if using.

Wild Rice Risotto with
Sweet Potatoes or Butternut Squash and Sage

Serves 4

PREP: 15 MINUTES
COOK: 45 MINUTES

1 cup water

$1/4$ cup wild rice, rinsed

2 tablespoons ghee, coconut oil, or olive oil

$1/2$ cup chopped leeks

$1/2$ cup short-grain rice (preferably arborio)

2 cups chicken broth, vegetable broth, Kombu Broth (page 190), or Ginger-Galangal Broth (page 191), warmed

$1/2$ cup peeled, cubed sweet potato or butternut squash

1 tablespoon nutritional yeast

1 teaspoon chopped fresh sage leaves

1 teaspoon coarse salt

$1/2$ teaspoon black pepper

1. Bring the water and wild rice to a boil in a small saucepan over high heat. Reduce heat to low, cover, and simmer for 45 minutes or until rice is tender. Drain the rice if necessary and set aside.

2. In a second saucepan, melt the ghee over medium heat, then add the leeks; cook until soft, stirring often. Add the short-grain rice and cook for three minutes, stirring constantly. Then add 1 cup of the warmed broth; simmer over medium-low heat for 10 minutes.

3. Stir in the remaining broth, sweet potato, and reserved wild rice. Cook until the rice and sweet potato are tender, 10 to 15 minutes, stirring occasionally to prevent sticking (add more broth if the rice gets dry before it's completely cooked through). Stir in the nutritional yeast, sage, salt, and black pepper.*

---

* Optional adaptogen: $1/2$ teaspoon astragalus root powder

Marinated Lentils

Serves 4 (³/₄ cup lentils each)

PREP: 10 MINUTES
COOK: 18 MINUTES

1¹/₂ cups black lentils

2 bay leaves

1¹/₄ teaspoons coarse salt

¹/₃ cup olive oil

2 teaspoons coriander seeds

1¹/₂ teaspoons fennel seeds

6 tablespoons chopped almonds

2 strips lemon peel

¹/₄ cup white wine vinegar

¹/₂ teaspoon coarse black pepper

1. In a large saucepan, combine the lentils and bay leaves. Add 3 cups water and the ¹/₂ teaspoon salt. Bring to a boil, covered, over medium heat. Reduce the heat and simmer, covered, until lentils are just tender, 15 to 20 minutes. Drain the lentils; remove and discard bay leaves.

2. In a small skillet, heat the oil over medium heat. Add the seeds, almonds, and lemon peel. Cook until the seeds are lightly toasted, about 3 minutes. Carefully remove the lemon peel. Pour the seasoned oil over the cooked lentils. Add the vinegar, the remaining ³/₄ teaspoon salt, and black pepper; stir to combine.

Tip: This recipe can be made up to 3 days ahead.

Coconut Collard Greens with Sweet Potatoes

Serves 4

PREP: 15 MINUTES
COOK: 1½ HOURS

1 pound collard greens, stemmed and chopped

1 yellow onion, thinly sliced

One 15-ounce can full-fat coconut milk

3 tablespoons honey, dark agave, or maple syrup

3 garlic cloves, minced

2 tablespoons grated peeled fresh ginger

1 teaspoon curry powder or garam masala

1 teaspoon coarse salt

½ teaspoon crushed red pepper

½ teaspoon freshly ground black pepper

½ teaspoon ground turmeric

¼ teaspoon ground allspice

¼ teaspoon ground cinnamon

1 medium (8-ounce) sweet potato, peeled and sliced into half-moons

Hot sauce to taste

1. To a large pot, add all of the ingredients except for the sweet potatoes and hot sauce. Add 3 to 4 cups of water and stir to combine.

2. Cover the pot with a tight-fitting lid and simmer the greens over medium heat, stirring occasionally, 1 hour 15 minutes. Add the sweet potatoes and cook, covered, until the sweet potatoes are tender and the collard greens are very tender, about 15 minutes more.

3. Serve the greens with hot sauce on the side.

New Potato and Pea Salad

Serves 4

PREP: 20 MINUTES
COOK: 20 MINUTES

1 pound red-skinned potatoes, halved or quartered if large

1 cup raw English peas or frozen peas

$1/2$ cup olive oil mayonnaise

$1/4$ cup chopped fresh dill or 2 tablespoons chopped fresh tarragon

3 tablespoons Dijon mustard

2 tablespoons minced shallot

1 tablespoon fresh lemon juice

1 teaspoon honey

1 teaspoon coarse salt

$1/2$ teaspoon black pepper

$1/2$ cup thinly sliced radishes

1. Boil the potatoes in a large pot over high heat in enough water to cover. Cook until just tender, adding the peas a few minutes before the potatoes are done. (If using frozen peas, do not cook with the potatoes.) Drain the potatoes and peas and spread out on a rimmed baking sheet to cool completely.

2. While the potatoes cool, in a large bowl whisk together the mayonnaise, herbs, mustard, shallot, lemon juice, honey, salt, and pepper. (If using frozen peas, add them to the bowl—do not thaw.) When the potatoes have cooled thoroughly, add them to the bowl with the radishes and toss gently to coat with dressing. Serve immediately or chill for up to 2 days.

Miso Broccoli

Serves 4

PREP: 10 MINUTES
COOK: 5 MINUTES

1 bunch broccoli, woody ends trimmed

2 tablespoons white miso

1 teaspoon honey or maple syrup

1 teaspoon coconut aminos

$^1/_2$ teaspoon rice vinegar

2 tablespoons extra-virgin olive oil

$^1/_2$ small red onion, cut into thin slivers

1 small clove garlic, thinly sliced

1 teaspoon toasted sesame oil

1 teaspoon sesame seeds, toasted

1. Cut the broccoli into florets and halve the stems lengthwise. Set aside. In a small bowl, stir together the miso, honey, coconut aminos, and vinegar. Set aside.

2. In a large skillet, heat the olive oil over medium-high heat. Add the onion and garlic and cook, stirring often, until softened, 1 to 2 minutes. Add the broccoli and cook, stirring often, until the broccoli is starting to brown, being careful not to burn the garlic, 2 to 3 minutes. Cover and cook until the broccoli is just tender, about 2 minutes. Add the miso mixture and stir to coat. Drizzle with sesame oil. Sprinkle with sesame seeds.

Kale Salad with Pistachio Vinaigrette

Serves 4

PREP: 10 MINUTES
BAKE: 8 MINUTES

1/2 cup shelled pistachios

1 large bunch curly kale, large stems trimmed and leaves roughly chopped

1/3 cup plus 2 teaspoons extra-virgin olive oil, divided

3 tablespoons champagne vinegar

1 tablespoon drained capers

2 teaspoons honey

1 clove garlic

Coarse salt

Freshly ground black pepper

1. Preheat the oven to 350°F. Place the pistachios on a large rimmed baking pan. Bake until lightly toasted, 8 to 10 minutes, stirring once halfway through. Let cool completely.

2. Meanwhile, place the kale in a large bowl; drizzle with 2 teaspoons of the olive oil. Gently massage the leaves until softened, 2 to 3 minutes.

3. In a food processor, process the pistachios, remaining olive oil, vinegar, capers, honey, and garlic until the nuts are finely chopped. Season to taste with salt and black pepper.

4. Pour the dressing over the kale and toss to coat.

DESERTS

Honey Grapefruit Sorbet

Serves 4

PREP: 15 MINUTES
FREEZE: 2 HOURS

1 cup fresh pink grapefruit juice, strained

¹/₂ cup water

¹/₃ cup honey (preferably orange blossom)

2 teaspoons minced grapefruit zest

Pinch of fine sea salt

1. Combine all the ingredients in a mixing bowl, stirring until honey dissolves. Transfer the mixture to an ice cream maker and churn according to manufacturer's instructions until sorbet is firm-slushy.

2. Scoop the mixture into a freezer-safe container and press a piece of waxed paper or parchment paper directly on the top before securing the lid. Freeze the sorbet until it's scoopable, about 2 hours.

Almond Berry Crumble

Serves 8

PREP: 20 MINUTES
COOK: 40 MINUTES

FOR THE FILLING

2 cups mixed fresh or frozen berries (such as blueberries, raspberries, blackberries, and/or strawberries)

1/4 cup pure maple syrup

2 teaspoons arrowroot

1 teaspoon pure vanilla extract

1/4 teaspoon ground nutmeg

FOR THE CRUMBLE

1 cup finely ground almond flour

1/2 cup gluten-free old-fashioned oats

1/2 cup unsweetened shredded coconut

1/2 teaspoon baking powder

1/2 teaspoon fine sea salt

6 tablespoons melted coconut oil or ghee

1/4 cup pure maple syrup

1/4 cup sliced almonds

1. Preheat the oven to 350°F. Coat a 9-inch round springform pan with nonstick cooking spray. In a large mixing bowl, toss together the berries, maple syrup, arrowroot, vanilla, and nutmeg. Set filling aside.

2. In a second bowl, combine the flour, oats, coconut, baking powder, and salt.* In a small bowl, stir together the melted coconut oil and 1/4 cup maple syrup. Add the liquid mixture to the dry ingredients and use your fingertips to mix until crumbly. Remove and reserve 1 cup of the crumb mixture, then pour the rest into the prepared pan. Press the mixture evenly over the bottom.

3. Pour the berry filling on top of the base, then sprinkle the reserved crumb mixture over the berries, followed by the sliced almonds. Bake the crumble for 40 minutes, or until the berries are bubbly and the crust is golden.

4. Cool the crumble for 10 minutes. Then carefully loosen the sides of the pan and remove. Let the crumble cool completely before cutting into wedges and serving.

---

* Optional adaptogen: 1/2 teaspoon moringa powder

Chocolate Pudding with Coconut Whipped Cream

Serves 6

PREP: 10 MINUTES
COOK: 10 MINUTES
CHILL: 2 HOURS TO OVERNIGHT

Two 15-ounce cans full-fat coconut milk

4 ounces good-quality unsweetened dark chocolate, chopped

¼ cup agave

Pinch of fine sea salt

Unsweetened cocoa powder (optional)

1. Pour 1 can of the coconut milk into a saucepan and warm it over medium heat. (Place the other can of coconut milk in the refrigerator.) When the milk begins to steam, remove the pan from the heat and add the chopped chocolate, agave, and salt. Let stand for 5 minutes to melt the chocolate. Then whisk until smooth and the chocolate is completely melted. Transfer pudding to a glass cup measure with a pour spout and divide evenly among six small ramekins or bowls. Cover and refrigerate the pudding until set, at least 2 hours, preferably overnight.

2. Before serving, scrape the solidified cream from the can of chilled coconut milk into a cold metal bowl. Beat with an electric mixer on medium-high speed until soft peaks form (tips curl). Spoon a small amount of coconut whipped cream on top of each pudding and sprinkle with unsweetened cocoa powder, if desired.

Deconstructed Apple Crisp

Serves 4

PREP: 10 MINUTES

BAKE: 15 MINUTES

2 Granny Smith or Gala apples, peeled if desired, halved and cored

1 tablespoon plus 2 teaspoons coconut oil, divided

$^1/_4$ cup unsalted whole almonds, coarsely chopped

$^1/_4$ cup unsalted shelled pistachios, coarsely chopped

$^1/_4$ cup shaved unsweetened coconut

$^1/_2$ teaspoon ground cinnamon

$^1/_4$ teaspoon ground coriander

Honey or pure maple syrup

1. Preheat the oven to 375°F. Place apples, cut side up, on an 8×8-inch baking pan. Drizzle with the 2 teaspoons coconut oil. Bake for 15 minutes or until tender.

2. Meanwhile, for the crisp, in a medium skillet, heat the remaining 1 tablespoon coconut oil over medium heat. Add the almonds and pistachios and cook, stirring often, for 2 minutes. Add the coconut and cook, stirring often, until the nuts and coconut are toasted. Sprinkle with the cinnamon and coriander.*

3. Place an apple half on each of 4 plates. Sprinkle with the crisp and drizzle with honey.

---

* Optional adaptogen: $^1/_2$ teaspoon maca powder

SNACKS

Filled Dates

Serves 4

START TO FINISH: 20 MINUTES

8 whole almonds

8 no-sugar-added dried apricots, halved

8 soft Medjool dates, pitted but left whole

$^{1}/_{2}$ cup almond butter, divided

$^{1}/_{2}$ cup unsweetened desiccated coconut

1. Stuff an almond and dried apricot piece inside the cavity of each pitted date.

2. Spread 2 teaspoons of the almond butter inside each date. Gently massage the date to help distribute the nut butter inside.

3. Spread the coconut onto a small plate. Roll the cut side of each date in the coconut to coat. Store in an airtight container at room temperature for up to 3 days.

Cinnamon-Scented Seed and Nut Granola with Goji Berries

Serves 10

PREP: 10 MINUTES
BAKE: 20 MINUTES
COOL: 15 MINUTES

1/4 cup ghee or coconut oil

2 tablespoons pure maple syrup

1 teaspoon ground cinnamon

1/2 teaspoon fine sea salt

1 cup chopped raw walnuts

1 cup sliced raw almonds

1 cup raw pepitas (green pumpkin seeds)

1 cup unsweetened coconut flakes

1/2 cup raw sunflower seeds

1/2 cup dried goji berries

1. Preheat the oven to 325°F. In a microwave, melt the ghee or coconut oil in a microwave-safe bowl with the maple syrup, cinnamon, and salt.* Add the walnuts, almonds, pepitas, coconut flakes, and sunflower seeds; toss to coat.

2. Spread the mixture evenly over a large parchment-lined rimmed sheet pan. Bake until the nuts are toasted and the mixture is dry, stirring two or three times during baking, 20 to 30 minutes.

3. Remove the granola from the oven and let cool completely before adding the goji berries. Store the granola in an airtight container for up to 1 week.

---

* Optional adaptogen: 1 teaspoon Siberian ginseng

Black Bean Hummus

Serve 8

START TO FINISH: 15 MINUTES

3 garlic cloves

1 jalapeño, seeded and chopped

$1/2$ cup natural peanut butter, almond butter, or tahini

$1/4$ cup fresh lime juice

Two 15-ounce cans black beans, drained and rinsed

1 teaspoon ground cumin

$1/2$ teaspoon ground coriander

$1/2$ teaspoon ground ancho chili powder or chili powder

$1/2$ teaspoon fine sea salt

Assorted cut-up fresh vegetables, such as cauliflower, carrots, and/or bell pepper strips

Sweet potato and/or plantain chips for dipping

1. In a food processor, pulse the garlic and jalapeño until minced. Add the peanut butter and lime juice and puree until smooth.

2. Add the drained black beans, spices, and salt. Puree until smooth, scraping the sides of the processor bowl periodically. If the hummus is too thick, drizzle in water, 1 tablespoon at a time, until the desired consistency is reached.

3. Store the hummus in the refrigerator in an airtight container for up to 5 days. Serve with assorted fresh vegetables and/or chips for dipping.

Crab-Salad-Stuffed Avocados

Serves 4 to 6

START TO FINISH: 15 MINUTES

1 pound lump crabmeat, coarsely flaked

³/₄ cup finely chopped celery

¹/₄ cup finely chopped red bell pepper

2 tablespoons finely chopped chives

2 tablespoons chopped fresh tarragon or flat-leaf parsley

3 tablespoons olive oil mayonnaise

1 tablespoon fresh lemon juice

2 teaspoons Dijon mustard

1 teaspoon coarse salt

¹/₂ teaspoon coarse black pepper

2 to 3 avocados, halved and pitted

Broccoli microgreens

1. In a medium bowl, gently fold together the crabmeat, celery, bell pepper, chives, and tarragon.

2. In a small bowl, stir together the mayonnaise, lemon juice, mustard, salt, and black pepper. Stir into the crabmeat mixture.

3. Spoon some of the crab salad onto each avocado half. Sprinkle with the microgreens.

Energy Bars

Serves 8

PREP: 30 MINUTES
BAKE: 10 MINUTES
CHILL: 30 MINUTES

1 cup gluten-free old-fashioned oats

1 cup raw walnuts, coarsely chopped

$^1/_4$ cup raw cashews

$^1/_4$ cup raw sunflower seeds

1 tablespoon flaxseed

1 tablespoon sesame seeds

$^1/_2$ cup golden raisins

$^1/_2$ cup chopped pitted Medjool dates

$^1/_2$ cup chopped dried apricots

$^1/_2$ cup natural nut butter (peanut, almond, cashew, etc.)

$^1/_2$ cup honey

2 tablespoons unsweetened cocoa powder

$^1/_4$ teaspoon fine sea salt

1. Preheat the oven to 375°F. Coat an 8×8-inch baking pan with nonstick spray. Spread the oats, walnuts, cashews, sunflower seeds, flaxseed, and sesame seeds on a rimmed sheet pan and toast in the oven for 10 to 15 minutes, stirring occasionally.

2. Transfer the toasted oat mixture to a large mixing bowl. Add the raisins, dates, and apricots; toss to combine. Melt the nut butter, honey, cocoa powder, and salt* in a small saucepan; when liquified, pour it over the oat mixture and stir to coat well.

3. Press the mixture evenly into the prepared pan. Refrigerate until firm, then cut into 8 bars. Store in an airtight container at room temperature or in the refrigerator for up to 1 week; freeze for up to 1 month (thaw at room temperature).

---

* Optional adaptogen: 1 teaspoon maca powder

CHAPTER 9

A Shameflammation-Free Life

I hope the last 21 days have been filled with self-discovery, reflection, and learning. If you've followed any of my other lifestyle plans, this book's plan probably felt very different. Some of you might feel like the plan was simple and easy to dive into and complete; for others, the feeling tasks may have pushed you outside your comfort zone. You may feel like an elimination diet was a walk in the park compared to the mindfulness exercises we completed in this plan.

What I hope you take away from the plan and this book is a more expansive perspective on physical and mental wellness. Over the last 21 days, we took steps to fuel ourselves, not just physically, but mentally, emotionally, and spiritually.

Whatever your experience was, I know you all have the same question: What's next? Well, this chapter is designed to answer that question and so much more.

Beyond the 21 Days

As I said before, this book is a little different from my others, but the truth is, they are all different facets of the same diamond of wellness—reflecting light in their own unique way but all a part of the same art of being well. If you're looking to continue with your wellness journey, I encourage you to take some time to reflect and think about which practices from the plan can be brought into your everyday life. Ask yourself: *What practices can help me prevent Shameflammation and feed my gut and my mind in equal measure?* Maybe it's setting daily boundaries with your phone, practicing meditation, taking a probiotic, flexible intermittent fasting, or even allowing yourself a good healthy cry every now and again. Make sure you tend to both the gut and the feeling elements because they are equally important to your overall health and wellness.

As you move out of the plan and back into your routine, I also encourage you to think about the following foundational features of the gut-feeling plan:

- Eating the foods that love you back and adapting these without judgment or guilt if your needs change.
- Making time to honor your emotional and psychological world, bringing in daily metaphysical meals, investing in this aspect of health as much as in food or exercise.
- Practicing radical self-compassion. You are your number one cheerleader, every step of the way.

Together, these three things make up the secret sauce of healthy and happy living in the long term. Yes, it really is as simple as that! My hope is that you continue coming back to this book, the plan, and the recipes when you need a reminder how important it is to slow down and care for yourself.

If you're looking to experiment more with your health and wellness, I recommend trying out the plans in some of my other books, too:

- *Intuitive Fasting.* I recommend this book for anyone looking to simplify their lifestyle, enhance overall wellness, promote longevity, and heal from metabolic conditions with mindful, flexible fasting.
- *The Inflammation Spectrum.* I recommend this book for any of you suffering from food sensitivities, an autoimmune condition, or another inflammation-based health problem.
- *Ketotarian.* I recommend this book for those looking to mix up their diet and celebrate the incredible (mostly) plant-based foods the earth has to offer for a fresh, Mediterranean spin on the ketogenic diet.

My other three books have more specific food plans, especially the elimination diet in *The Inflammation Spectrum*. You can feel free to try one, do them all, and come back to the 21-Day Gut-Feeling Plan whenever you feel like your body and brain could use some time and attention. I also talk about all of these topics on my podcast *The Art of Being Well*. If you feel like you need an even more tailored approach to food or would like comprehensive labs and functional medicine guidance for your specific health goals, go to www.drwillcole.com to learn about my telehealth center.

Food Peace and Body Peace

Throughout this book, I've given you the tools you need to start living a life free of Shameflammation. I'm sure many of you were visualizing a life in which your emotional health is so optimal that it never affects your physical health, where you tackle stress completely, and perpetually live in the present moment. But here's the catch—there's no such thing. Why? Because humans aren't capable of perfection, and the human body is both inherently flawed and inherently wonderful, all at the same time.

When something goes awry with our health or our happiness, which will inevitably happen for all of us at one point or another, the only way out is acceptance and self-compassion. We have to allow ourselves the space to be human. Otherwise we start to blame ourselves for every little misstep or thing that goes wrong. And where there's blame, there's shame. I see patients all the time who feel flawed or lacking. Why? Because they want to obtain this unreachable standard of waking up every day feeling flawless, energized, and happy. It's all just way too much to live up to, isn't it?

In this book, we consistently challenged the idea that if we just do enough—if we just complete that cleanse, eat all the right things, and do the hardest workouts—we'll achieve optimal health and happiness. As much of a fan as I am of a good cleanse or an exercise class, a healthy gut-feeling connection isn't just about ticking things off a list. In fact, I'd argue that one of the most important parts of restoring a healthy gut-feeling connection was the time we spent focused on doing less. Instead of more doing, we focused more on being. Self-sabotaging behavior is a by-product of not knowing our intrinsic worth. Owners of luxury cars don't need to be told to take great care in how they fuel, clean, drive, and park their valuable vehicle. On the other hand, a driver of an old rusted, decrepit car may not care as much if it gets beat up a little more. Many of us don't believe that we are worthy of good things; we are convinced there is something about us that is inherently unlovable. Knowing that you are a Lamborghini and not a jalopy changes everything. Awareness that you are a valuable creation who is worthy of wellness is the path to food peace and body peace, a catalyst for sustainable healing. It's not about behavior modification, shaming your way to wellness. The paradigm shift is realizing that self-care is a form of self-respect. This book is your proverbial pause to discover what's in alignment with how you want to feel and what is not—a deep remembering of who you were created to be.

The journey to healing is the journey home to yourself, wholly. By consistently implementing the practices in this book, you will continue to make peace with the broken pieces while simultaneously creating the space to heal them. Repairing your gut-feeling connection is the end of the war between your body and food. This is where you will find food peace and body peace. And remember, you don't have to have it all together or have it all figured out to start improving your health and how you feel. Health can still happen, rough edges and all.

Inner resistance, shame, and disdain for the parts of you that you feel are unacceptable can disrupt that delicate gut-feeling connection and sabotage your health journey. Be easy on yourself. Radical acceptance is just that: *radical*. Nourishing your body and spirit with foods and acts of stillness is a way to take your power back. Healing yourself is an act of rebellion, culturally; an act of empowerment, personally. Getting healthy on your own terms, like any act of agency, free thought, and free will, is a revolutionary act today. But undoubtedly, peace comes from nourishing vibrant wellness.

As you continue to heal your gut-feeling connection, you will stop fighting reality, stop responding with impulsive or destructive behaviors, and let go of bitterness or shame. I see people do this every day, ordinary people finding extraordinary new levels of deep wellness, rising from the ashes of what no longer serves them. I want the same for you. In truth, you are the greatest masterpiece you will ever work on. This, my friend, is your art of being well.

NOTES

◇◇◇◇◇◇◇◇

Chapter 1. As Above, So Below

1. Thomas C. Neylan and Aoife O'Donovan, "Inflammation and PTSD." *PTSD Research Quarterly* 29, no. 4 (2019); https://www.ptsd.va.gov/publications/rq_docs/V29N4.pdf.

2. Fahimeh Haghighatdoost, Awat Feizi, Ahmad Esmaillzadeh, et al., "Drinking Plain Water Is Associated with Decreased Risk of Depression and Anxiety in Adults: Results from a Large Cross-Sectional Study." *World Journal of Psychiatry* 8, no. 3 (2018): 88–96; doi: 10.5498/wjp.v8.i3.88.

3. Supa Pengpid and Karl Peltzer, "High Sedentary Behaviour and Low Physical Activity Are Associated with Anxiety and Depression in Myanmar and Vietnam." *International Journal of Environmental Research and Public Health* 16, no. 7 (2019): 1251; doi: 10.3390/ijerph16071251.

4. Brené Brown, "Shame Is Lethal." SuperSoul Sunday, OWN, March 24, 2013; https://www.youtube.com/watch?v=GEBjNv5M784.

5. Luna Dolezal and Barry Lyons, "Health-Related Shame: An Affective Determinant of Health." *Medical Humanities* 43, no. 3 (2017): 257–63; doi: 10.1136/medhum-2017-011186.

6. Juliana G. Breines, Myriam V. Thoma, Danielle Gianferante, et al., "Self-Compassion as a Predictor of Interleukin-6 Response to Acute Psychosocial Stress." *Brain, Behavior, and Immunity* 37 (2014): 109–14; doi: 10.1016/j.bbi.2013.11.006.

Chapter 2. Gut

1. John B. Furness, Brid P. Callaghan, Leni R. Rivera, and Hyun-Jung Cho, "The Enteric Nervous System and Gastrointestinal Innervation: Integrated Local and Central Control." *Advances in Experimental Medicine and Biology* 817 (2014): 39–71; doi: 10.1007/978-1-4939-0897-4_3.

2. Tatenda A. Mudyanadzo, Chandanbindya Hauzaree, Oksana Yerokhina, et al., "Irritable Bowel Syndrome and Depression: A Shared Pathogenesis." *Cureus* 10, no. 8 (2018): e3178; doi: 10.7759/cureus.3178.

3. Charles Darwin, *The Expression of the Emotions in Man and Animals* (New York: D. Appleton, 1897), 69.

4. Adi Aran, Maya Eylon, Moria Harel, et al., "Lower Circulating Endocannabinoid Levels in Children with Autism Spectrum Disorder." *Molecular Autism* 10, no. 2 (2019): 2. doi: 10.1186/s13229-019-0256-6.

5. Ethan B. Russo, "Clinical Endocannabinoid Deficiency Reconsidered: Current Research Supports the Theory in Migraine, Fibromyalgia, Irritable Bowel, and Other Treatment-Resistant Syndromes." *Cannabis and Cannabinoid Research* 1, no. 1 (2016): 154–65; doi: 10.1089/can.2016.0009.

6. Amar Sarkar, Soili M. Lehto, Siobhán Harty, et al., "Psychobiotics and the Manipulation of Bacteria-Gut-Brain Signals." *Trends in Neuroscience* 39, no. 11 (2016): 763–81; doi: 10.1016/j.tins.2016.09.002.

7. Monique Aucoin, Laura LaChance, Umadevi Naidoo, et al., "Diet and Anxiety: A Scoping Review." *Nutrients* 13, no. 12 (2021): 4418; doi: 10.3390/nu13124418.

8. Satu Immonen, Jyrki Launes, Ilkka Järvinen, et al., "Moderate Alcohol Use Is Associated with Decreased Brain Volume in Early Middle Age in Both Sexes." *Scientific Reports* 10, no. 1 (2020): 13998; doi: 10.1038/s41598-020-70910-5.

9. Joshua P. Smith and Carrie L. Randall, "Anxiety and Alcohol Use Disorders: Comorbidity and Treatment Considerations." *Alcohol Research: Current Reviews* 34, no. 4 (2012): 414–31; PMCID: PMC3860396.

10. Anna Ford, "How 'Dry January' Is the Secret to Better Sleep, Saving Money and Losing Weight." University of Sussex, January 2, 2019; https://www.sussex.ac.uk/news/article/47131-how-dry-january-is-the-secret-to-better-sleep-saving-money-and-losing-weight.

11. Karen M. Davison, Shen Lamson Lin, Hongmei Tong, et al., "Nutritional Factors, Physical Health and Immigrant Status Are Associated with Anxiety Disorders among Middle-Aged and Older Adults: Findings from Baseline Data of the Canadian Longitudinal Study on Aging (CLSA)." *International Journal of Environmental Research and Public Health* 17, no. 5 (2020): 1493; doi: 10.3390/ijerph17051493; University of Toronto, "Low Fruit and Vegetable Intakes and Higher Body Fat Linked to Anxiety Disorders." EurekAlert! February 27, 2020; https://www.eurekalert.org/news-releases/889635.

12. Felice N. Jacka, Adrienne O'Neil, Rachelle Opie, et al., "A Randomised Controlled Trial of Dietary Improvement for Adults with Major Depression (the 'SMILES' Trial)." *BMC Medicine* 15, no. 1 (2017): 23; doi: 10.1186/s12916-017-0791-y.

13. Rachel Feltman, "The Gut's Microbiome Changes Rapidly with Diet." *Scientific American*, December 14, 2013; https://www.scientificamerican.com/article/the-guts-microbiome-changes-diet/.

Chapter 3. Feelings

1. Michael Ashworth, "Can Stress Cause Death?" PsychCentral, June 29, 2022; https://psychcentral.com/stress/is-stress-the-number-one-killer.

2. Nicholas A. Cummings and Gary R. VandenBos, "The Twenty Years Kaiser-Permanente Experience with Psychotherapy and Medical Utilization: Implications for National Health Policy and National Health Insurance." *Health Policy Quarterly* 1, no. 2 (1981): 159–75.

3. National Institute for Occupational Safety and Health, "STRESS . . . At Work." Centers for Disease Control and Prevention, October 7, 2020; https://www.cdc.gov/niosh/docs/99-101/default.html.

4. Vivek Pillai, Thomas Roth, Heather M. Mullins, and Christopher L. Drake, "Moderators and Mediators of the Relationship Between Stress and Insomnia: Stressor Chronicity, Cognitive Intrusion, and Coping." *Sleep* 37, no. 7 (2014): 1199–1208A; doi: 10.5665/sleep.3838.

5. Rajita Sinha and Ania M. Jastreboff, "Stress as a Common Risk Factor for Obesity and Addiction." *Biological Psychiatry* 73, no. 9 (2013): 827–35; doi: 10.1016/j.biopsych.2013.01.032.

6. Boonsong Ongphiphadhanakul, Shi Lieh Fang, Kam-Tsun Tang, et al., "Tumor Necrosis Factor-Alpha Decreases Thyrotropin-Induced 5'-Deiodinase Activity in FRTL-5 Thyroid Cells." *European Journal of Endocrinology* 130, no. 5 (1994): 502–7; doi: 10.1530/eje.0.1300502.

7. Nicholas J. Justice, "The Relationship Between Stress and Alzheimer's Disease." *Neurobiology of Stress* 8 (2018): 127–33; doi: 10.1016/j.ynstr.2018.04.002.

8. Nicole D. Powell, Erika K. Sloan, Michael T. Bailey, and Steven W. Cole, "Social Stress Up-Regulates Inflammatory Gene Expression in the Leukocyte Transcriptome Via β-Adrenergic Induction of Myelopoiesis." *Proceedings of the National Academy of Sciences of the USA* 110, no. 41 (2013): 16574–579; doi: 10.1073/pnas.1310655110.

9. Elizabeth Mostofsky, Malcolm Maclure, Jane B. Sherwood, et al., "Risk of Acute Myocardial Infarction After the Death of a Significant Person in One's Life: The Determinants of Myocardial Infarction Onset Study." *Circulation* 125, no. 3 (2012): 491–96; doi: 10.1161/CIRCULATIONAHA.111.061770.

10. Elizabeth Mostofsky, "Beth Israel Study: You Can Die of a Broken Heart." *Boston Business Journal,* January 9, 2012; https://www.bizjournals.com/boston/news/2012/01/09/beth-israel-it-is-possible-to-die-of.html.

11. Mihaela-Luminiţa Staicu and Mihaela Cuţov, "Anger and Health Risk Behaviors." *Journal of Medicine and Life* 3, no. 4 (2010): 372–75; PMCID: PMC3019061.

12. Sherita Hill Golden, Janice E. Williams, Daniel E. Ford, et al., "Anger Temperament Is Modestly Associated with the Risk of Type 2 Diabetes Mellitus: The Atherosclerosis Risk in Communities Study." *Psychoneuroendocrinology* 31, no. 3 (2006): 325–32; doi: 10.1016/j.psyneuen.2005.08.008.

13. Yára Dadalti Fragoso, Erika Oliveira da Silva, and Alessandro Finkelsztejn, "Correlation Between Fatigue and Self-Esteem in Patients with Multiple Sclerosis." *Arquivos de Neuro-Psiquiatria* 67, no. 3B (2009): 818–21; doi: 10.1590/s0004-282x2009000500007.

14. Vincent J. Felitti, Robert F. Anda, Dale Nordenberg, et al., "Relationship of Childhood Abuse and Household Dysfunction to Many of the Leading Causes of Death in Adults. The Adverse Childhood Experiences (ACE) Study." *American Journal of Preventive Medicine* 14, no. 4 (1998): 245–58; doi: 10.1016/s0749-3797(98)00017-8.

15. Shanta R. Dube, DeLisa Fairweather, William S. Pearson, et al., "Cumulative Childhood Stress and Autoimmune Diseases in Adults." *Psychosomatic Medicine* 71, no. 2 (2009): 243–50; doi: 10.1097/PSY.0b013e3181907888.

16. Brent Bezo and Stefania Maggi, "Living in 'Survival Mode': Intergenerational Transmission of Trauma from the Holodomor Genocide of 1932–1933 in Ukraine." *Social Science & Medicine* 134 (2015): 87–94; doi: 10.1016/j.socscimed.2015.04.009.

17. Tori Rodriguez, "Descendants of Holocaust Survivors Have Altered Stress Hormones." *Scientific American*, March 1, 2015; https://www.scientificamerican.com/article/descendants-of-holocaust-survivors-have-altered-stress-hormones/.

18. Lingshu Zhang, Pingying Qing, Hang Yang, et al., "Gut Microbiome and Metabolites in Systemic Lupus Erythematosus: Link, Mechanisms and Intervention." *Frontiers in Immunology* 12 (2021): 686501; doi: 10.3389/fimmu.2021.686501.

19. Sergey Yegorov, Dimitriy Babenko, Samat Kozhakhmetov, et al., "Psoriasis Is Associated with Elevated Gut IL-1α and Intestinal Microbiome Alterations." *Frontiers in Immunology* 11 (2020): 571319; doi: 10.3389/fimmu.2020.571319.

20. Odelya Gertel Kraybill, "PTSD May Be a Risk Factor for Autoimmune Disease." *Psychology Today*, February 28, 2020; https://psychologytoday.com/us/blog/expressive-trauma-integration/202002/ptsd-may-be-risk-factor-autoimmune-disease.

21. Deborah Boggs Bookwalter, Kimberly A. Roenfeldt, Cynthia A. LeardMann, et al., "Posttraumatic Stress Disorder and Risk of Selected Autoimmune Diseases Among US Military Personnel." *BMC Psychiatry* 20, no. 1 (2020): 23; doi: 10.1186/s12888-020-2432-9.

22. Cohen Veterans Network, "America's Mental Health 2018." Published online October 10, 2018; https://www.cohenveteransnetwork.org/wp-content/uploads/2018/10/Research-Summary-10-10-2018.pdf.

23. John Weeks, "IFM Survey Teases Characteristics of Functional Medicine Practice." *Integrative Practitioner*, August 19, 2016; https://www.integrativepractitioner.com/practice-management/news/ifm-survey-teases-on-characteristics-of-functional-medicine-practice.

24. National Institute of Mental Health, Mental Health Information Statistics, https://www.nimh.nih.gov/health/statistics/prevalence/any-mental-illness-ami-among-us-adults.shtml. Centers for Disease Control and Prevention Morbidity and Mortality Weekly Report, https://www.cdc.gov/mmwr/volumes/66/wr/mm6630a6.htm. C. Pritchard, A. Mayers, and D. Baldwin, "Changing Patterns of Neurological Mortality in the 10 Major Developed Countries—1979–2010," *Public Health* 127, no. 4 (2013): 357–68; doi: 10.1016/j.puhe.2012.12.018.

25. J. M. Twenge, "The Age of Anxiety? The Birth Cohort Change in Anxiety and Neuroticism, 1952–1993." *Journal of Personality and Social Psychology,* 79, no. 6 (2000): 1007–21; https://doi.org/10.1037/0022-3514.79.6.1007.

26. Barbara Starfield, "Is US Health Really the Best in the World?" *JAMA* 284, no. 4 (2000): 483–85; doi: 10.1001/jama.284.4.483.

27. Jason Lazarou, Bruce H. Pomeranz, and Paul N. Corey, "Incidence of Adverse Drug Reactions in Hospitalized Patients: A Meta-Analysis of Prospective Studies." *JAMA* 279, no. 15 (1998): 1200–205; doi: 10.1001/jama.279.15.1200.

Chapter 4. Is Shameflammation Sabotaging Your Health?

1. World Health Organization, "WHO Reveals Leading Causes of Death and Disability Worldwide: 2000–2019." News release, December 9, 2020; https://www.who.int/news/item/09-12-2020-who-reveals-leading-causes-of-death-and-disability-worldwide-2000-2019.

2. Centers for Disease Control and Prevention, "National Diabetes Statistics Report." https://www.cdc.gov/diabetes/basics/prediabetes.html#:~:text=Approximately%2096%20million%20American%20adults,%2C%20heart%20disease%2C%20and%20stroke.

3. Nielson T. Baxter, Nicholas A. Lesniak, Hamide Sinani, et al., "The Glucoamylase Inhibitor Acarbose Has a Diet-Dependent and Reversible Effect on the Murine Gut Microbiome." *mSphere* 4, no. 1 (2019): e00528-18; doi: 10.1128/mSphere.00528-18.

4. Samuel J. Kallus and Lawrence J. Brandt, "The Intestinal Microbiota and Obesity." *Journal of Clinical Gastroenterology* 46, no. 1 (2012): 16–24; doi: 10.1097/MCG.0b013e31823711fd.

5. Jotham Suez, Tal Korem, David Zeevi, et al., "Artificial Sweeteners Induce Glucose Intolerance by Altering the Gut Microbiota." *Nature* 514 (2014): 181–86; doi: 10.1038/nature13793.

6. American Thyroid Association, "General Information/Press Room," March 13, 2012; https://www.thyroid.org/media-main/press-room/.

7. Dominika Berent, Krzysztof Zboralski, Agata Orzechowska, and Piotr Gałecki, "Thyroid Hormones Association with Depression Severity and Clinical Outcome in Patients with Major Depressive Disorder." *Molecular Biology Reports* 41, no. 4 (2014): 2419–25; doi: 10.1007/s11033-014-3097-6.

8. Agathocles Tsatsoulis, "The Role of Stress in the Clinical Expression of Thyroid Autoimmunity." *Annals of the New York Academy of Sciences* 1088 (2006): 382–95; doi: 10.1196/annals.1366.015.

9. Olga Yaylali, Suna Kiraç, Mustafa Yilmaz, et al., "Does Hypothyroidism Affect Gastrointestinal Motility?" *Gastroenterology Research and Practice* 2009 (2009): 529802; doi: 10.1155/2009/529802.

10. Andrew E. Rosselot, Christian I. Hong, and Sean R. Moore, "Rhythm and Bugs: Circadian Clocks, Gut Microbiota, and Enteric Infections." *Current Opinion in Gastroenterology* 32, no. 1 (2016): 7–11; doi: 10.1097/MOG.0000000000000227.

11. Gosia Lipinska, Beth Stuart, Kevin G. F. Thomas, et al., "Preferential Consolidation of Emotional Memory During Sleep: A Meta-Analysis." *Frontiers in Psychology* 10 (2019): 1014; doi: 10.3389/fpsyg.2019.01014.

12. Erik Schéle, Louise Grahnemo, Fredrik Anesten et al., "The Gut Microbiota Reduces Leptin Sensitivity and the Expression of the Obesity-Suppressing Neuropeptides Proglucagon (*Gcg*) and Brain-Derived Neurotrophic Factor (*Bdnf*) in the Central Nervous System." *Endocrinology* 154, no. 10 (2013): 3643–51; doi: 10.1210/en.2012-2151.

13. Lisa M. Jaremka, Martha A. Belury, Rebecca R. Andridge, et al. "Interpersonal Stressors Predict Ghrelin and Leptin Levels in Women." *Psychoneuroendocrinology* 48 (2014): 178–88; doi: 10.1016/j.psyneuen.2014.06.018.

Chapter 5. Feed Your Gut and Your Brain

1. Kelly M. Adams, Martin Kohlmeier, and Steven H. Zeisel, "Nutrition Education in U.S. Medical Schools: Latest Update of a National Survey." *Academic Medicine* 85, no. 9 (2010): 1537–42; doi: 10.1097/ACM.0b013e3181eab71b.

2. Marigold Castillo, Ronald Feinstein, James Tsang, and Martin Fisher, "Basic Nutrition Knowledge of Recent Medical Graduates Entering a Pediatric Residency Program." *International Journal of Adolescent Medicine and Health* 28, no. 4 (2016): 357–61; doi: 10.1515/ijamh-2015-0019.

3. Agnès Le Port, Alice Gueguen, Emmanuelle Kesse-Guyot, et al. "Association Between Dietary Patterns and Depressive Symptoms over Time: A 10-Year Follow-Up Study of the GAZEL Cohort." *PLoS One* 7, no. 12 (2012): e51593; doi: 10.1371/journal.pone.0051593.

4. David Mischoulon, "Omega-3 Fatty Acids for Mood Disorders." Harvard Health, October 27, 2020; https://www.health.harvard.edu/blog/omega-3-fatty-acids-for-mood-disorders-2018080314414.

5. Elisabetta Lauretti and Domenico Praticò, "Effect of Canola Oil Consumption on Memory, Synapse and Neuropathology in the Triple Transgenic Mouse Model of Alzheimer's Disease." *Scientific Reports 71,* no. 1 (2017): 17134; doi: 10.1038/s41598-017-17373-3.

6. Irwin J. Schatz, Kamal Masaki, Katsuhiko Yano, et al., "Cholesterol and All-Cause Mortality in Elderly People from the Honolulu Heart Program: A Cohort Study." *Lancet* 358, no. 9279 (2001): P351–55; doi: 10.1016/S0140-6736(01)05553-2.

7. MedlinePlus Medical Encyclopedia, "Facts About Trans Fats," National Library of Medicine, https://medlineplus.gov/ency/patientinstructions/000786.htm.

8. Dominika Głąbska, Dominika Guzek, Barbara Groele, and Krystyna Gutkowska, "Fruit and Vegetable Intake and Mental Health in Adults: A Systematic Review." *Nutrients* 12, no. 1 (2020): 115; doi: 10.3390/nu12010115.

9. Simone Radavelli-Bagatini, Lauren C. Blekkenhorst, Marc Sim, et al., "Fruit and Vegetable Intake Is Inversely Associated with Perceived Stress Across the Adult Lifespan." *Clinical Nutrition* 40, no. 5 (2021): 2860–67; doi: 10.1016/j.clnu.2021.03.043.

10. Natalia S. Klimenko, Alexander V. Tyakht, Anna S. Popenko, et al., "Microbiome Responses to an Uncontrolled Short-Term Diet Intervention in the Frame of the Citizen Science Project." *Nutrients* 10, no. 5 (2018): 576; doi:10.3390/nu10050576.

Chapter 6. Feed Your Head and Your Heart

1. George M. Slavich and Michael R. Irwin, "From Stress to Inflammation and Major Depressive Disorder: A Social Signal Transduction Theory of Depression." *Psychological Bulletin* 140, no. 3 (2014): 774–815; doi: 10.1037/a0035302.

2. Hans Kirschner, Willem Kuyken, Kim Wright, et al., "Soothing Your Heart and Feeling Connected: A New Experimental Paradigm to Study the Benefits of Self-Compassion." *Clinical Psychological Science* 7, no. 3 (2019): 545–65; doi: 10.1177/2167702618812438.

3. Emiliano Ricciardi, Giuseppina Rota, Lorenzo Sani, et al., "How the Brain Heals Emotional Wounds: The Functional Neuroanatomy of Forgiveness." *Frontiers in Human Neuroscience* 7 (2013): 839; doi: 10.3389/fnhum.2013.00839.

4. Bessel van der Kolk, *The Body Keeps the Score: Brain, Mind, and Body in the Healing of Trauma* (New York: Penguin, 2015), 283.

5. Madhav Goyal, Sonal Singh, Erica M. S. Sibinga, et al., "Meditation Programs for Psychological Stress and Well-Being: A Systematic Review and Meta-Analysis." *JAMA Internal Medicine* 174, no. 3 (2014): 357–68; doi:10.1001/jamainternmed.2013.13018.

6. "Meditation and Mindfulness: What You Need to Know." National Center for Complementary and Integrative Health, https://www.nccih.nih.gov/health/meditation -and-mindfulness-what-you-need-to-know.

7. Jenna E. Boyd, Ruth A. Lanius, and Margaret C. McKinnon, "Mindfulness-Based Treatments for Posttraumatic Stress Disorder: A Review of the Treatment Literature and Neurobiological Evidence." *Journal of Psychiatry and Neuroscience* 43, no. 1 (2018): 7–25; doi: 10.1503/jpn.170021.

8. Laurie Keefer and E. B. Blanchard, "A One Year Follow-Up of Relaxation Response Meditation as a Treatment for Irritable Bowel Syndrome." *Behaviour Research and Therapy* 40, no. 5 (2002): 541–46; doi: 10.1016/s0005-7967(01)00065-1.

9. Rongxiang Tang, Karl J. Friston, and Yi-Yuan Tang, "Brief Mindfulness Meditation Induces Gray Matter Changes in a Brain Hub." *Neural Plasticity* 2020 (2020): 8830005; doi: 10.1155/2020/8830005.

10. Jordan Fallis, "How to Stimulate Your Vagus Nerve for Better Mental Health," April 24, 2022, originally published January 21, 2017; https://www.optimallivingdynamics.com/ blog/how-to-stimulate-your-vagus-nerve-for-better-mental-health-brain-vns-ways -treatment-activate-natural-foods-depression-anxiety-stress-heart-rate-variability-yoga -massage-vagal-tone-dysfunction.

11. Pratibha Pradip Pandekar and Poovishnu Devi Thangavelu, "Effect of 4-7-8 Breathing Technique on Anxiety and Depression in Moderate Chronic Obstructive Pulmonary Disease Patients." *International Journal of Health Sciences and Research* 9, no. 5 (2019): 209–17; https://www.ijhsr.org/IJHSR_Vol.9_Issue.5_May2019/32.pdf.

12. Liza Varvogli and Christina Darviri, "Stress Management Techniques: Evidence-Based Procedures That Reduce Stress and Promote Health." *Health Science Journal* 5, no. 2 (2011): 74–89; https://www.inmed.us/wp-content/uploads/7-Stress-Management-Techniques-Evidence-Based-Procedures-that-Reduce-Stress-and-Promote-Health.-Health-Science-Journal-2011.pdf.

13. Xiao Ma, Zi-Qi Yue, Zhu-Qing Gong, et al., "The Effect of Diaphragmatic Breathing on Attention, Negative Affect and Stress in Healthy Adults." *Frontiers in Psychology* 8 (2017): 874; doi: 10.3389/fpsyg.2017.00874.

14. Marlysa B. Sullivan, Matt Erb, Laura Schmalzl, et al., "Yoga Therapy and Polyvagal Theory: The Convergence of Traditional Wisdom and Contemporary Neuroscience for Self-Regulation and Resilience." *Frontiers in Human Neuroscience* 12 (2018): 67; doi: 10.3389/fnhum.2018.00067.

15. Agnieszka Golec de Zavala, Dorottya Lantos, and Deborah Bowden, "Yoga Poses Increase Subjective Energy and State Self-Esteem in Comparison to 'Power Poses.'" *Frontiers in Psychology* 8 (2017): 752; doi: 10.3389/fpsyg.2017.00752.

16. Jocelyn N. García-Sesnich, Mauricio Garrido Flores, Marcela Hernández Ríos, and Jorge Gamonal Aravena, "Longitudinal and Immediate Effect of Kundalini Yoga on Salivary Levels of Cortisol and Activity of Alpha-Amylase and Its Effect on Perceived Stress." *International Journal of Yoga* 10, no. 2 (2017): 73–80; doi: 10.4103/ijoy.IJOY_45_16.

17. Kimberley Luu and Peter A. Hall, "Examining the Acute Effects of Hatha Yoga and Mindfulness Meditation on Executive Function and Mood." *Mindfulness* 8, no. 4 (2017): 873–80; doi: 10.1007/s12671-016-0661-2.

18. Anup Sharma, Marna S. Barrett, Andrew J. Cucchiara, et al., "A Breathing-Based Meditation Intervention for Patients with Major Depressive Disorder Following Inadequate Response to Antidepressants: A Randomized Pilot Study." *Journal of Clinical Psychiatry* 78, no. 1 (2017): e59–e63; doi: 10.4088/JCP.16m10819.

19. Mayo Clinic Staff, "Tai Chi: A Gentle Way to Fight Stress." Mayo Clinic, February 26, 2021; https://www.mayoclinic.org/healthy-lifestyle/stress-management/in-depth/tai-chi/art-20045184

20. Sarosh J. Motivala, John Sollers, Julian Thayer, and Michael R. Irwin, "Tai Chi Chih Acutely Decreases Sympathetic Nervous System Activity in Older Adults." *Journals of Gerontology: Series A* 61, no. 11 (2006): 1177–80; doi: 10.1093/gerona/61.11.1177.

21. Tonny Elmose Andersen, Yael Lahav, Hanne Ellegaard, and Claus Manniche, "A Randomized Controlled Trial of Brief Somatic Experiencing for Chronic Low Back Pain and Comorbid Post-Traumatic Stress Disorder Symptoms." *European Journal of Psychotraumatology* 8, no. 1 (2017): 1331108; doi: 10.1080/20008198.2017.1331108.

22. José Alexandre S. Crippa, Guilherme Nogueira Derenusson, Thiago Borduqui Ferrari, et al., "Neural Basis of Anxiolytic Effects of Cannabidiol (CBD) in Generalized Social Anxiety Disorder: A Preliminary Report." *Journal of Psychopharmacology* 25, no. 1 (2011): 121–30; doi: 10.1177/0269881110379283.

23. Matthew N. Hill and Sachin Patel, "Translational Evidence for the Involvement of the Endocannabinoid System in Stress-Related Psychiatric Illnesses." *Biology of Mood and Anxiety Disorders* 3, no. 1 (2013): 19; doi: 10.1186/2045-5380-3-19.

24. Alline C. Campos, Zaira Ortega, Javier Palazuelos, et al., "The Anxiolytic Effect of Cannabidiol on Chronically Stressed Mice Depends on Hippocampal Neurogenesis: Involvement of the Endocannabinoid System." *International Journal of Neuropsychopharmacology* 16, no. 6 (2013): 1407–19; doi: 10.1017/S1461145712001502.

Chapter 7. The 21-Day Gut-Feeling Plan

1. James Clear, *Atomic Habits: An Easy & Proven Way to Build Good Habits & Break Bad Ones* (New York: Avery, 2018), 25.

2. Joanna Rymaszewska, David Ramsey, and Sylwia Chładzińska-Kiejna, "Whole-Body Cryotherapy as Adjunct Treatment of Depressive and Anxiety Disorders." *Archivum Immunologiae et Therapie Experimentalis (Warsz)* 56, no. 1 (2008): 63–68. doi: 10.1007/s00005-008-0006-5.

3. Erik M. Olsson, Bo von Schéele, Alexander G. Panossian, "A Randomised, Double-Blind, Placebo-Controlled, Parallel-Group Study of the Standardised Extract SHR-5 of the Roots of *Rhodiola rosea* in the Treatment of Subjects with Stress-Related Fatigue." *Planta Medica* 75, no. 2 (2009): 105–12; doi: 10.1055/s-0028-1088346.

4. Q. G. Chen, Y. S. Zeng, Z. Q. Qu, et al., "The Effects of *Rhodiola rosea* Extract on 5-HT Level, Cell Proliferation and Quantity of Neurons at Cerebral Hippocampus of Depressive Rats." *Phytomedicine* 16, no. 9 (2009): 830–38; doi: 10.1016/j.phymed.2009.03.011.

5. Marc Maurice Cohen, "Tulsi—*Ocimum sanctum*: A Herb for All Reasons." *Journal of Ayurveda and Integrative Medicine* 5, no. 4 (2014): 251–59; doi: 10.4103/0975-9476.146554.

6. Mayumi Nagano, Kuniyoshi Shimizu, Ryuichiro Kondo, et al., "Reduction of Depression and Anxiety by 4 Weeks *Hericium erinaceus* Intake." *Biomedical Research* 31, no. 4 (2010): 231–37; doi: 10.2220/biomedres.31.231.

7. Deepak Langade, Subodh Kanchi, Jaising Salve, et al., "Efficacy and Safety of Ashwagandha (*Withania somnifera*) Root Extract in Insomnia and Anxiety: A Double-Blind, Randomized, Placebo-Controlled Study." *Cureus* 11, no. 9 (2019): e5797; doi: 10.7759/cureus.5797.

8. Christoph A. Thaiss, David Zeevi, Maayan Levy, et al., "Transkingdom Control of Microbiota Diurnal Oscillations Promotes Metabolic Homeostasis." *Cell* 159, no. 3 (2014): 514–29; doi: 10.1016/j.cell.2014.09.048.

9. Jiffin K. Paulose, John M. Wright, Akruti G. Patel, and Vincent M. Cassone, "Human Gut Bacteria Are Sensitive to Melatonin and Express Endogenous Circadian Rhythmicity." *PLoS One* 11, no. 1 (2016): e0146643; doi: 10.1371/journal.pone.0146643.

10. Laura I. Hazlett, Mona Moieni, Michael R. Irwin, et al., "Exploring Neural Mechanisms of the Health Benefits of Gratitude in Women: A Randomized Controlled Trial." *Brain, Behavior, and Immunity* 95 (2021): 444–53; doi: 10.1016/j.bbi.2021.04.019.

11. Alex M. Wood, Stephen Joseph, Joanna Lloyd, and Samuel Atkins, "Gratitude Influences Sleep Through the Mechanism of Pre-Sleep Cognitions." *Journal of Psychosomatic Research* 66, no. 1 (2009): 43–48; doi: 10.1016/j.jpsychores.2008.09.002.

12. American Heart Association News, "Could Sunshine Lower Blood Pressure? Study Offers Enlightenment." February 28, 2020, https://www.heart.org/en/news/2020/02/28/could-sunshine-lower-blood-pressure-study-offers-enlightenment.

13. Alan C. Geller, Nina G. Jablonski, Sherry L. Pagoto, et al., "Interdisciplinary Perspectives on Sun Safety." *JAMA Dermatology* 154, no. 1 (2018): 88–92; doi: 10.1001/jamadermatol.2017.4201.

14. Akinori Masuda, Takashi Kihara, Tsuyoshi Fukudome, et al., "The Effects of Repeated Thermal Therapy for Two Patients with Chronic Fatigue Syndrome." *Journal of Psychosomatic Research* 58, no. 4 (2005): 383–87; doi: 10.1016/j.jpsychores.2004.11.005.

15. Tanjaniina Laukkanen, Jari A. Laukkanen, and Setor K. Kunutsor, "Sauna Bathing and Risk of Psychotic Disorders: A Prospective Cohort Study." *Medical Principles and Practice* 27, no. 6 (2018): 562–69; doi: 10.1159/000493392.

16. Taryn Luntz, "U.S. Drinking Water Widely Contaminated." *Scientific American*, December 14, 2009; https://www.scientificamerican.com/article/tap-drinking-water-contaminants-pollutants/.

17. Elmar Wienecke and Claudia Nolden, "Langzeit-HRV-Analyse zeigt Stressreduktion durch Magnesiumzufuhr" [Long-Term HRV Analysis Shows Stress Reduction by Magnesium Intake]. *MMW Fortschritte der Medizin* 158, suppl. 6 (2016): 12–16; doi: 10.1007/s15006-016-9054-7.

18. Danny Phelan, Patricio Molero, Miguel A. Martínez-González, and Marc Molendijk, "Magnesium and Mood Disorders: Systematic Review and Meta-Analysis." *BJPsych Open* 4, no. 4 (2018): 167–79; doi: 10.1192/bjo.2018.22.

19. Asmir Gračanin, Lauren M. Bylsma, and Ad J. J. M. Vingerhoets, "Is Crying a Self-Soothing Behavior?" *Frontiers in Psychology* 5 (2014): 502; doi: 10.3389/fpsyg.2014.00502.

20. Juan Murube, "Hypotheses on the Development of Psychoemotional Tearing." *The Ocular Surface* 7, no. 4 (2009): 171–75; doi: 10.1016/s1542-0124(12)70184-2.

21. Ruth Ann Atchley, David L. Strayer, and Paul Atchley, "Creativity in the Wild: Improving Creative Reasoning Through Immersion in Natural Settings." *PLoS One* 7, no. 12 (2012): e51474; doi: 10.1371/journal.pone.0051474.

22. Margaret M. Hansen, Reo Jones, and Kirsten Tocchini, "Shinrin-Yoku (Forest Bathing) and Nature Therapy: A State-of-the-Art Review." *International Journal of Environmental Research and Public Health* 14, no. 8 (2017): 851; doi: 10.3390/ijerph14080851.

23. Qing Li, "Effect of Forest Bathing Trips on Human Immune Function." *Environmental Health and Preventive Medicine* 15, no. 1 (2010): 9–17; doi: 10.1007/s12199-008-0068-3.

24. Ibid.

25. Department of Economic and Social Affairs, United Nations, "2018 Revision of World Urbanization Prospects," May 16, 2018. https://www.un.org/development/desa/publications/2018-revision-of-world-urbanization-prospects.html#:~:text=Today%2C%2055%25%20of%20the%20world's,increase%20to%2068%25%20by%202050.

26. Catherine E. Milner and Kimberly A. Cote, "Benefits of Napping in Healthy Adults: Impact of Nap Length, Time of Day, Age, and Experience with Napping." *Journal of Sleep Research* 18, no. 2 (2009): 272–81; doi: 10.1111/j.1365-2869.2008.00718.x.

27. Jennifer R. Goldschmied, Philip Cheng, Kathryn Kemp, et al., "Napping to Modulate Frustration and Impulsivity: A Pilot Study." *Personality and Individual Differences* 86 (2015): 164–67; doi: 10.1016/j.paid.2015.06.013.

28. Sanae Oriyama, Yukiko Miyakoshi, and Toshio Kobayashi, "Effects of Two 15-min Naps on the Subjective Sleepiness, Fatigue and Heart Rate Variability of Night Shift Nurses." *Industrial Health* 52, no. 1 (2014): 25–35; doi: 10.2486/indhealth.2013-0043.

29. Madhukar H. Trivedi, Tracy L. Greer, Timothy S. Church, et al., "Exercise as an Augmentation Treatment for Nonremitted Major Depressive Disorder: A Randomized, Parallel Dose Comparison." *Journal of Clinical Psychiatry* 72, no. 5 (2011): 677–84; doi: 10.4088/JCP.10m06743.

ACKNOWLEDGMENTS

Amber, Solomon, and Shiloh: "I will love you until time itself is done, and so long as you are by my side, I am well pleased with the world."

My team: You are my family and my closest friends. Thank you for your consistent devotion, diligence, and compassion for our patients and for one another.

My patients around the world: Thank you for letting me be a part of your sacred journey into wellness. I do not take that responsibility lightly. Serving you is truly an honor.

Heather, Diana, Michele, and everyone at Rodale and Waterbury: You are the best literary team I could have dreamed of. Thank you for always listening to my vision and doing everything to help it come to life.

Gretchen: Thank you for your friendship and putting your heart into this book with me.

Gwyneth: The first person who I told what I wanted this book to say. You are a true friend. Thank you for your deep kindness and always championing me.

Kiki and my goop family: I am immensely grateful for you. Thank you for your years of friendship and giving me a voice.

Elle Macpherson, Dr. Alejandro Junger, Melissa Urban, Dr. Josh Axe, Jason and Colleen Wachob: Thank you for your friendship, support, guidance, and personal and professional advice over the years in this space of wellness.

Finally, thank you to everyone in the functional medicine and wellness world: Continue being a light in the darkness.

INDEX

Index

Index

237

sugar cravings, 17, 56, 116–17
suicide, 52
sun exposure, 125, 130–31
supplements
    for sleep, 125
    Vitamin D, 131–32
sweet potatoes
    Coconut Collard Greens with Sweet Potatoes,
        200
    Sweet Potato and Mushroom Pancakes, 161
    Sweet Potato "Toasts" with Avocado, 156
    Wild Rice Risotto with Sweet Potatoes and
        Sage, 198
sympathetic nervous system. *See* nervous system
    function; stress

Tacos, Beef-Poblano Cabbage, 188
tai chi, 97
Tempeh Hash, 172
Thai-Style Chicken Larb, 165
Thai-Style Chicken Stir-Fry, 187
therapy, 4, 87–89
thyroid function and problems, 39, 59–60
Tofu and Kimchi, Jarred Spicy Ramen Noodles
    with, 189
Tom Kha, Vegan, 192
toxic productivity, 41, 66
toxic relationships, 66, 100–102
toxins and detoxification, 64–67
trans fats, 76
trauma, 24, 43–46, 48. *See also* PTSD
    physical health and, 3, 23, 43, 45, 49–50, 58
    sleep and, 62–63
    therapies for, 87–89, 97–98

tulsi, 122
tuna
    Cajun Tuna Salad with Chickpeas, 169
    Chickpea Penne Puttanesca with Tuna,
        182
Turkey Sausage, Quiche Muffins with Broccoli
    and, 157
21-Day Gut-Feeling Plan. *See* Gut-Feeling Plan,
    21-Day

ulcerative colitis, 32, 39

vagus nerve and vagal tone, 25–26, 28, 91, 97,
    124
    polyvagal theory, 46–48, 96
van der Kolk, Bessel, 50, 91
Vegan Tom Kha, 192
vegetables and fruits, 73–74, 77, 78–80. *See also*
    specific types
Vitamin D, 130–32

water, 2–3, 135–37
weight gain, 39. *See also* obesity/overweight
Wheel of Emotions, 113, *114*
Wild Rice Risotto with Sweet Potatoes or
    Butternut Squash and Sage, 198
wraps
    Curried Lentil Wraps with Coconut-Lime
        Yogurt Sauce, 168
    Korean-Inspired Beef Wraps with Kimchi
        and Ginger-Sesame Mayo, 177

yeast overgrowth, 2, 19, 31
yoga, 95, 96

ABOUT THE AUTHOR

DR. WILL COLE, IFMCP, DNM, DC, is a leading functional medicine expert who consults with people around the world, having started one of the first functional medicine telehealth centers. Named one of the top fifty functional medicine and integrative doctors in the nation, Dr. Cole specializes in clinically investigating underlying factors of chronic disease and customizing a functional medicine approach for thyroid issues, autoimmune conditions, hormonal imbalances, digestive disorders, and brain problems. He is the host of *The Art of Being Well* podcast and author of *Ketotarian, The Inflammation Spectrum,* and the *New York Times* bestseller *Intuitive Fasting.* To learn more and connect with him on social media, visit drwillcole.com.

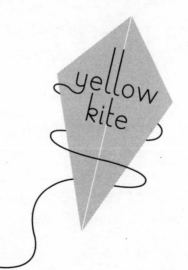

books to help you live a good life

Join the conversation and tell
us how you live a #goodlife

🐦 @yellowkitebooks
📘 YellowKiteBooks
📌 Yellow Kite Books
📷 YellowKiteBooks